High Cholesterol

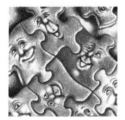

what you should know

**Blackwell
Science**

High Cholesterol

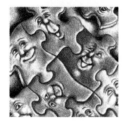

what you should know

NEW HANOVER COUNTY
PUBLIC LIBRARY
201 CHESTNUT STREET
WILMINGTON, NC 28401

Written by Dean J. Kereiakes, MD, FACC,
and Douglas Wetherill, MS
Illustrated by Laura L. Seeley

©2001 by Robertson & Fisher Publishing Company. Second Edition.

Written by: Dean J. Kereiakes, MD, FACC; and Douglas Wetherill, MS
Contributing Editors: Paul Ribisl, PhD; Rona Wharton, MEd, RD, LD; Charles J. Glueck, MD, PhD;
                     and Nancy Bulach-Kolb
Illustrated by: Laura L. Seeley

Distributors:
Blackwell Publishing
c/o AIDC
P.O. Box 20, 50 Winter Sport Lane, Williston, VT 05495-0020 USA
(Telephone orders: 800-216-2522; fax orders: 802-864-7626)

Blackwell Science, Ltd.
c/o Marston Book Services, Ltd.
P.O. Box 269, Abingdon, Oxon OX14 4YN, England
(Telephone orders: 44-01235-465500; fax orders: 44-01235-465555)

All rights reserved. No part of this book may be reproduced in any form or by any means without
permission in writing from the publisher, except by a reviewer who may quote brief passages in a review.

Printed in Canada
01 02 03 04 5 4 3 2 1 (ISBN:0-632-04533-7)

The Blackwell Science logo is a trademark of Blackwell Science Ltd., registered at the United Kingdom
Trade Marks Registry.

A catalog record for this book is available from the U.S. Library of Congress.

To Janette, Marcy, Nancy, and the program participants. Thanks for all your support and encouragement.

— Douglas

The authors are truly indebted to these people for their technical assistance: Peggy Marquette, Janette Weisbrodt, Lynne Haag, Angela Ginty, Richard Hunt, Phil Sexton, and Sara Dumford.

Treatment Disclaimer

This book is for education purposes, not for use in the treatment of medical conditions. It is based on skilled medical opinion as of the date of publication. However, medical science advances and changes rapidly. Furthermore, diagnosis and treatment are often complex and involve more than one disease process or medical issue to determine proper care. If you believe you may have a medical condition described in the book, consult your doctor.

Table of Contents

Introduction

In the past, there was little need for a book devoted solely to cholesterol control because the life expectancy of Americans was only 47 years of age — and coronary heart disease was not a leading cause of death.

However, our standard of living has improved substantially. Our technological advances have created both a sedentary lifestyle and a diet that is characterized by overabundance. Consequently, we have a disproportionate prevalence of cardiovascular disease and an increasing incidence of diabetes.

Currently, more than 97 million people in the United States have cholesterol levels greater than 200 mg/dL. High serum cholesterol is the leading precursor of all forms of cardiovascular disease. This book explains how cholesterol is useful to the body. It also explains how too much cholesterol can damage the body and produce serious health consequences.

This book does not replace the need for discussing your medical condition with your doctor. Please remember, your doctor will know how to help you manage your cholesterol and other risk factors for coronary heart disease.

— Dean and Douglas

About Cholesterol

High cholesterol

Cardiovascular disease generally develops as a result of poor lifestyle habits combined with inherited disorders. Behaviors that increase our chances of developing heart disease are called **risk factors**.

High cholesterol is a major risk factor for heart disease. Currently, more than **97 million** Americans have cholesterol levels greater than **200 mg/dL**, thereby increasing their risk of developing heart disease.

By controlling **cholesterol** levels and other risk factors, you can potentially reduce the chance of having a cardiac event. Please remember, it is important that you discuss **your** specific medical history with your doctor.

Risk Factors

What are the risk factors for cardiovascular disease? They include:

1) Elevated cholesterol
2) Smoking
3) Diabetes
4) Hypertension
5) Obesity
6) Age
7) Family history
8) Physical inactivity

4

1. Elevated cholesterol

A small amount of **cholesterol** is good for our bodies. Like a piece of a puzzle, cholesterol fits into our lives by serving many useful purposes in our bodies.

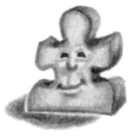

CHOLESTEROL

Cholesterol is a "waxlike substance" that serves as a "building block" within the **cell membrane**.

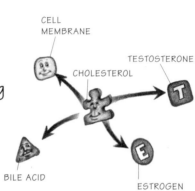

CELL MEMBRANE

TESTOSTERONE

CHOLESTEROL

BILE ACID

ESTROGEN

Cholesterol is also used to make **hormones,** especially those found in reproduction: **estrogen** and **testosterone**.

Cholesterol is used to make **bile acids** that help break down fat in our intestines.

6

Cholesterol has other functions in the body. **Vitamin D** is made when the body absorbs sunlight in skin and combines it with a form of cholesterol. Vitamin D is needed to absorb calcium into the body.

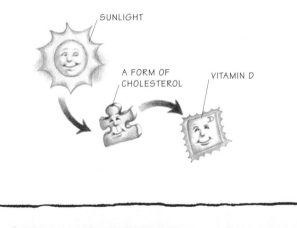

SUNLIGHT

A FORM OF CHOLESTEROL

VITAMIN D

Excessive sun exposure may be harmful, but 30 minutes a day is effective in producing sufficient amounts of vitamin D provided that skin is exposed to natural, outdoor sunlight. People who live in northern climates of the United States may not achieve adequate sunlight exposure. Contact your doctor to find out if you should take vitamin D supplements.

Where does cholesterol come from?

About two-thirds of all the cholesterol in the body is produced by the **liver**.

LIVER

STOMACH

GALLBLADDER

9

The remaining one-third of the body's cholesterol is absorbed by the **digestive system** from the foods we eat.

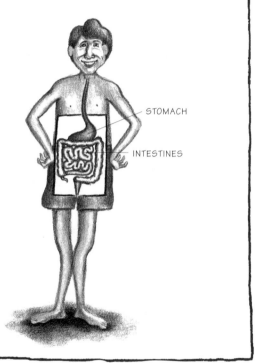

STOMACH

INTESTINES

Foods that contain cholesterol are those that come from animal products. Sources of cholesterol include chicken, eggs, beef, and dairy products. Foods, especially those high in **saturated fat**, can influence the total cholesterol.

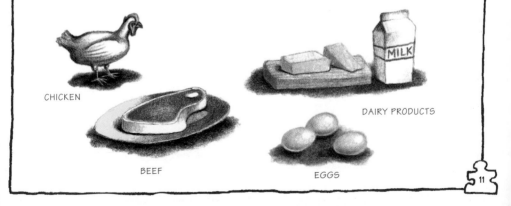

CHICKEN

BEEF

EGGS

DAIRY PRODUCTS

How does cholesterol move throughout the body?

Once **cholesterol** and **trigylcerides** are digested, they are packaged into bundles that carry them to the different parts of the body. **Cholesterol** is used to build cell walls and is used in hormone production. **Triglycerides** are fat molecules that provide energy for the body. Both **cholesterol** and **triglycerides** are carried through the blood by **lipoproteins**.

CHOLESTEROL

TRIGLYCERIDES

Lipoproteins (lipids)

The 5 major classes of lipoproteins are: **chylomicrons, VLDL-cholesterol, IDL-cholesterol, LDL-cholesterol, and HDL-cholesterol.**

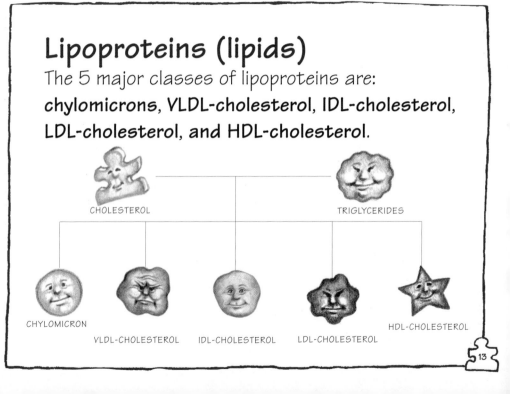

CHOLESTEROL

TRIGLYCERIDES

CHYLOMICRON

VLDL-CHOLESTEROL

IDL-CHOLESTEROL

LDL-CHOLESTEROL

HDL-CHOLESTEROL

CHYLOMICRONS

Chylomicrons are composed mainly of triglycerides and some cholesterol.

VLDL-cholesterol (very low density lipoprotein) carries cholesterol from the liver.

VLDL-CHOLESTEROL

IDL-CHOLESTEROL

IDL-cholesterol (intermediate density lipoprotein) is made from VLDL-cholesterol and carries cholesterol through the blood.

LDL-cholesterol
(low-density lipoprotein) is
the "bad" cholesterol.
It often binds to the inside
of the artery wall.

LDL-CHOLESTEROL

HDL-CHOLESTEROL

HDL-cholesterol
(high-density lipoprotein)
is the "good" cholesterol.
It removes LDL-cholesterol
from the blood.

Total cholesterol is defined as the total amount of cholesterol in **ALL** the **lipoproteins** circulating in the blood.

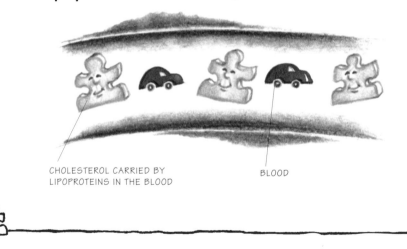

CHOLESTEROL CARRIED BY
LIPOPROTEINS IN THE BLOOD

BLOOD

2. What about smoking?

Don't do it. Smoking is bad for the entire cardiovascular system because it:

A) Introduces carbon monoxide into the body

B) Lowers the "good" HDL-cholesterol

A. Carbon monoxide

Oxygen attaches to the red blood cells in the lungs. Red blood cells transport the oxygen throughout the body.

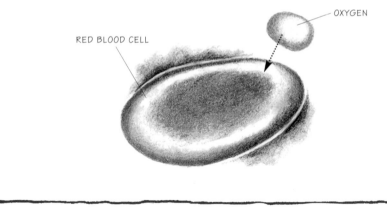

OXYGEN

RED BLOOD CELL

When you smoke, you inhale carbon monoxide into your lungs. Carbon monoxide binds to the red blood cells at the site where oxygen normally binds.

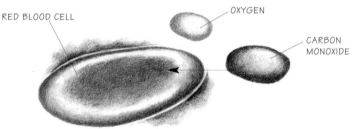

RED BLOOD CELL

OXYGEN

CARBON MONOXIDE

Therefore, less oxygen is carried by the blood, resulting in less oxygen available for use in the heart, muscles, and throughout the body. People who smoke may have abnormal heartbeats as well.

Understandably, smoking has harmful effects, especially for anyone who has already had a heart attack or bypass surgery. More importantly, there is an increased likelihood of a second heart attack or need for another bypass surgery if you continue to smoke after an initial cardiac incident.

Smoking is also a risk factor for peripheral vascular disease (blockages of the arteries to the brain, kidneys and legs).

B. Lower HDL-cholesterol

Two other reasons for not smoking are that it reduces the amount of HDL-cholesterol or "good cholesterol" in your bloodstream, and it makes your blood clot more easily, increasing the potential for an arterial blockage (heart attack or stroke).

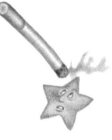

SMOKING
REDUCES
HDL-CHOLESTEROL

21

3. Diabetes

What exactly is diabetes? The working cells need sugar for energy. Sugar is absorbed through the digestive system after a meal or snack. **Insulin** is released by the **pancreas** to allow the body to use sugar as a source of nutrition and energy. That may be hard to visualize. This may help ...

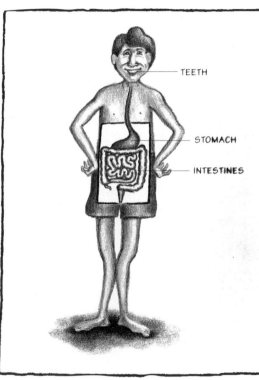

TEETH

STOMACH

INTESTINES

While you eat, the digestive system (teeth, stomach, and intestines) breaks your food down into smaller particles that are used by your body.

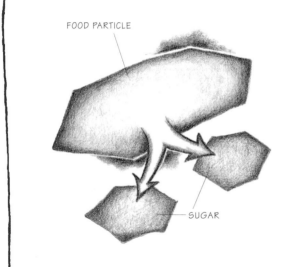

FOOD PARTICLE

SUGAR

Some food is broken down into particles of **sugar**. Sometimes this sugar is referred to as **carbohydrates** or **glucose**.

24

Sugar moves from the digestive system to the blood and travels throughout the body to feed the working cells. The sugar is the energy packet the cells need to do work like running and breathing.

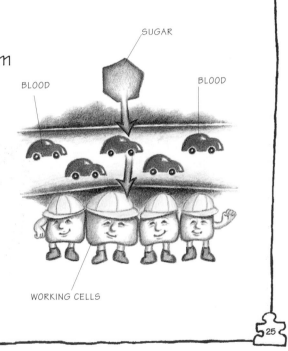

SUGAR

BLOOD

BLOOD

WORKING CELLS

At the same time, the body sends a signal to the **pancreas** telling it to release **insulin** into the bloodstream.

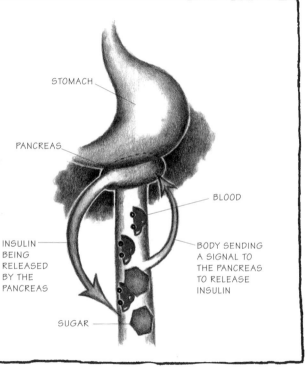

STOMACH

PANCREAS

BLOOD

INSULIN BEING RELEASED BY THE PANCREAS

BODY SENDING A SIGNAL TO THE PANCREAS TO RELEASE INSULIN

SUGAR

Insulin acts like a **key** that unlocks the doors of the cells to let sugar move in. The working cells can then use the sugar for energy to do their jobs. This is how your body uses sugar. However ...

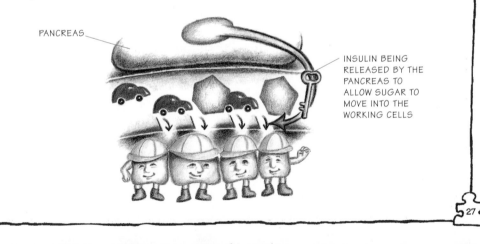

PANCREAS

INSULIN BEING RELEASED BY THE PANCREAS TO ALLOW SUGAR TO MOVE INTO THE WORKING CELLS

Without the key (insulin), the sugar cannot get out of the bloodstream and into the working cells. The sugar builds up in the blood, and the working cells get hungry. This is what happens in diabetes. A diabetic's body cannot move sugar from the blood into the cells.

Diabetes is a major risk factor for cardiovascular disease. Approximately 80% of diabetic patients eventually die of cardiovascular disease. It has been estimated that 50% of diabetics have some form of coronary heart disease prior to being diagnosed with diabetes.

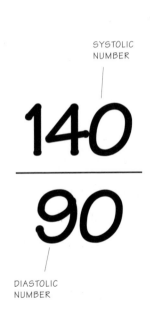

SYSTOLIC NUMBER

140
———
90

DIASTOLIC NUMBER

4. Hypertension

Hypertension is commonly referred to as high blood pressure. If you have a **systolic pressure** greater than 140 mm Hg and/or a **diastolic pressure** greater than 90 mm Hg on 2 separate visits to the doctor, then you may have high blood pressure.

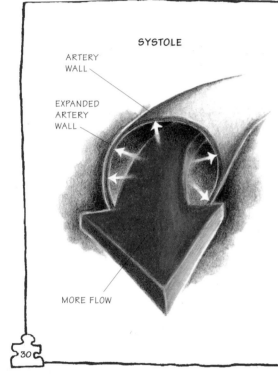

SYSTOLE

ARTERY WALL

EXPANDED ARTERY WALL

MORE FLOW

What is **systolic pressure**? Blood comes out of the heart in 1 big thrust. The artery expands to handle the blood. The amount of pressure put on the expanded artery wall is called **systolic pressure**.

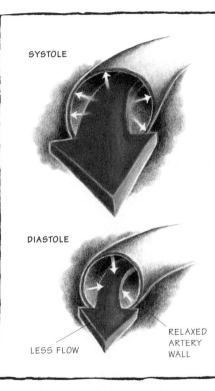

SYSTOLE

DIASTOLE

LESS FLOW

RELAXED
ARTERY
WALL

After the artery expands during systole, it relaxes back to its normal size. It is similar to a rubber band that goes back to its normal shape after being stretched. Normal pressure on the artery wall during relaxation is called **diastolic pressure**.

How does hypertension relate
to cardiovascular disease?

Blood pressure is a result of the blood flowing through the artery (cardiac output) and the resistance of the artery wall (vascular resistance). If that sounds too technical, here ... this may help:

Blood pressure = Cardiac output x vascular resistance

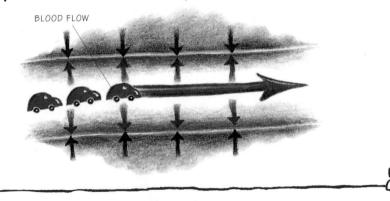

BLOOD FLOW

If a lot of resistance is created by either the blood or the artery wall, then there is more pressure as the blood travels through the artery. If it takes more energy to get the blood through the arteries, then your heart has to work harder with each beat. Most people with high blood pressure do not realize they have it. No wonder hypertension is called the "silent killer."

What contributes to hypertension?

Several factors may contribute to hypertension
and cardiovascular disease. These include:

> Excess dietary salt
> Excess alcohol intake
> Stress
> Age
> Genetics and family history
> Obesity
> Physical inactivity
> High saturated fat diet

Salt

Salt helps conserve water in your body. The American Heart Association Step II Diet recommends that the average person consume no more than 2,400 mg of salt per day, especially those individuals who are salt sensitive. Excess dietary salt may contribute to both hypertension and to your body retaining too much water.

If you are retaining too much water, then you are increasing your blood volume (cars) without adding space. This increase will result in more pressure in the arteries.

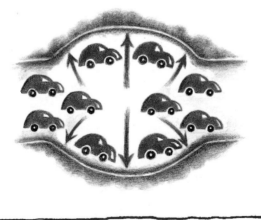

Alcohol consumption

A common concern for individuals who are at risk for cardiovascular disease is alcohol consumption — mainly because there seems to be conflicting evidence about the benefits versus the risks of drinking. Experts agree that excess alcohol consumption over time can lead to many harmful effects, including high blood pressure, cirrhosis of the liver, and damage to the heart. The issue is the balance between **moderate** and **excessive** alcohol consumption.

While the evidence shows that there is a protective effect for moderate alcohol consumption, this benefit disappears with excessive intake. Men should consume no more than 2 drinks* daily, and women, because of their smaller body size, should not consume more than 1 drink* each day. The 7 to 14 allowable drinks in a week should not be consumed in a few days or during a weekend of binge drinking.

*A guide: One drink is defined as 5 ounces of wine, 12 ounces of beer, or 1-1/2 ounces of 80-proof liquor.

People who should not drink include individuals with high levels of triglycerides in their blood (over 300 mg/dL), women who are pregnant, individuals who are under age, people with a genetic predisposition for alcoholism or who are recovering from alcoholism, and those taking certain medications.

What about stress?

When you are under stress, your brain releases signals to the body through the nerves. These signals allow your body to respond to various situations.

Arteries have nerves attached to them. The nerves can either cause the arteries to relax or can put more tension on the walls of the arteries. If you are under a lot of stress, the nerves send signals to tighten or narrow the arteries.

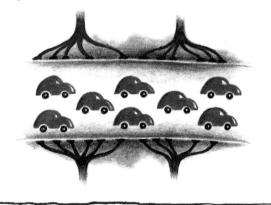

Narrowing the artery is like taking away a lane of traffic. There is still the same number of cars (blood) with less space (artery). This increases the pressure inside the artery.

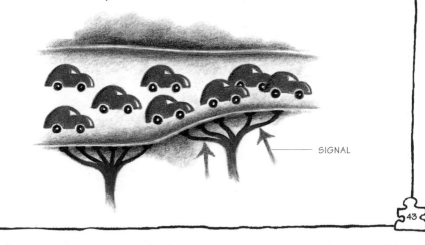

SIGNAL

So,

something you can do to improve your blood pressure is reduce stress. You can accomplish this by practicing meditation, doing deep breathing exercises, or doing exercise, such as going for a walk, riding a bike, or taking a swim.

5. Obesity

The American Heart Association has described obesity as a major risk factor for cardiovascular disease. What exactly is obesity?

Metropolitan Life's height/weight tables are often used to determine a recommended weight for an individual based on age and gender. Generally, those who are 20% over the recommended weight for their height are considered to be overweight — but not necessarily obese. Obesity refers to fatness rather than weight. Men who have greater than 25% of their body weight as fat and women who have more than 35% are considered to be obese. Obesity and being overweight carry significant health risks, are directly related to cardiovascular risk factors, and may:

1) raise triglycerides (a "bad" blood fat)
2) lower HDL-cholesterol (the "good" cholesterol)
3) raise LDL-cholesterol (the "bad" cholesterol)
4) raise blood pressure and
5) increase the risk of developing diabetes

Obesity may be related to both genetics (nature) and lifestyle (nurture). Generally speaking, obesity occurs when the calories we consume exceed the calories we burn through activities of daily living and exercise. We store the excess calories as fat reserves, thus contributing to obesity and ultimately increasing the risk of coronary disease. Obesity has increased in men and women in every decade over the past 50 years. There is a misconception that Americans are overeating and eating too much fat. In fact, as a nation we are eating less fat, fewer calories, and still gaining weight — primarily due to the lower levels of physical activity in our youth and adult lives. A sedentary lifestyle could be the real culprit.

6. Age

Aging has an effect on the risk of cardiovascular disease because aging causes changes in the heart and blood vessels. As people age, they become less active, gain more weight, and the effects of a sedentary lifestyle, smoking, and poor diet continue to damage the heart and circulation by increasing blood pressure and cholesterol levels. Blood pressure increases with aging, in part because arteries gradually lose some of their elasticity and, over time, may not be as resilient.

7. Family history

A **family history** of cardiovascular disease could reflect genetics and/or an unhealthy family lifestyle. If most of your family members smoke, are sedentary, and have a poor diet — then these are harmful habits that increase the risk of heart disease in your family. However, unlike your genes, these behaviors can be changed.

On the other hand, if your family has a healthful lifestyle but there is still a high incidence of cardiovascular disease, then it is likely that genetics is playing a role. We are learning more about the importance of genetic risk for vascular disease. In the future, treatment may be tailored to an individual's own genetic makeup. In either case, by practicing a healthful lifestyle, you can help reduce your risk rather than giving up and thinking you have no control over your destiny.

If you have a strong family history of heart disease, you should talk to your doctor about how to monitor your child's cholesterol at an earlier age.

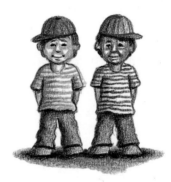

Why children?

Compared with the rest of the industrialized world, the United States has a much greater proportion of children with high cholesterol.

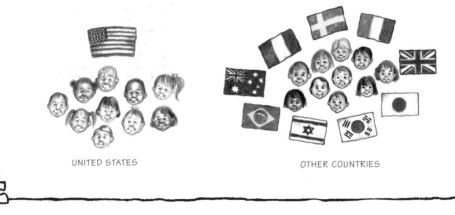

UNITED STATES   OTHER COUNTRIES

When should my child's total cholesterol be tested?

If both parents have high cholesterol, or if one parent has had a cardiac event (heart attack or bypass surgery at a very early age — before age 40), then their child should have his or her total cholesterol tested at age 2. Your doctor will help you to determine the frequency of testing.

What are some treatment options for lowering my child's cholesterol?

Generally speaking, the first sensible option for parents is to modify their child's diet. A registered dietitian can provide suggestions for making your child's diet healthier.

Are there any other treatment options that may help improve my child's cholesterol?

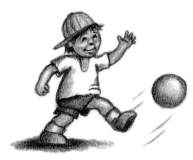

Encourage your child to get plenty of exercise. Exercise does not necessarily change the total cholesterol, but it can increase the HDL-cholesterol or "good" cholesterol. This habit will be helpful throughout his or her life.

Children are not the only ones to benefit from exercise. Lack of exercise is a risk factor for adults, too ...

8. Physical inactivity

Lack of exercise is a major contributor to obesity, diabetes, and hypertension. Beginning an exercise program may help you feel better, help you have more energy, help you lose some weight, lower your cholesterol, lower your blood pressure, help you look better, and improve your muscle tone. Also, beginning an exercise routine can increase your HDL-cholesterol or "good cholesterol" — especially if exercise is associated with weight loss.

Having a high **HDL-cholesterol** level is a "positive" factor. An HDL-cholesterol of greater than 60 mg/dL helps to reduce your risk of having cardiovascular disease.

For most people, the best way to naturally increase HDL-cholesterol is through **aerobic exercise** and **losing excess fat**. Always follow your doctor's recommendation when starting an exercise program.

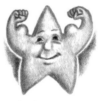

INCREASE HDL-CHOLESTEROL WITH EXERCISE AND FAT LOSS

How Does Cholesterol Damage an Artery?

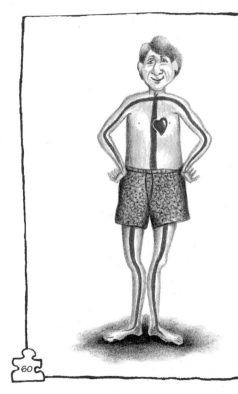

Arteries and veins

Arteries and veins wind throughout the body carrying blood. Arteries carry blood away from the heart. Veins carry blood back to the heart.

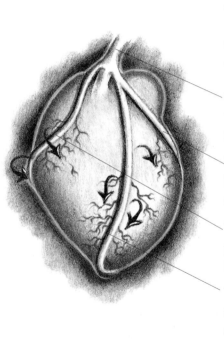

The heart has its own arteries to provide blood to the heart muscle.

The **aorta** supplies blood to the arteries of the heart as well as to the rest of the body.

The **circumflex artery** supplies blood to the lateral or side aspect of the heart.

The **right coronary artery** provides blood to the back or underside of the heart.

The **left anterior descending artery** supplies blood to the front of the heart.

61

To give you some idea of their size, the **coronary arteries** are only about the size of a strand of spaghetti.

(APPROXIMATE SIZE OF SPAGHETTI)

At birth, the inside of the arteries, including the coronary arteries, is slippery — similar to a nonstick pan. The blood cells (represented by the small cars) flow smoothly through the arteries.

BLOOD

62

What happens to an artery during a person's lifetime?

Fatty streaks in the arteries start to develop in the first decade of life as a result of lipids moving into the cell wall of the artery.

LIPIDS MOVING INTO THE ARTERY WALL

These fatty streaks may become more advanced **atherosclerotic lesions** in the presence of risk factors such as smoking, high blood pressure, obesity, high cholesterol, and physical inactivity. The fatty streaks may then progress to **atheromas** and **fibroatheromas**, which are more "advanced lesions" and are often referred to as **plaque**.

ATHEROSCLEROTIC LESION

BLOOD FLOW

Buildups may occur at different points along the length of the artery. Plaque buildups are not limited to the arteries of the heart. They can occur and restrict blood flow in arteries throughout your body.

PLAQUE BUILDUP

Plaque restricts the flow of blood through the artery, similar to orange construction barrels you have seen on the highway. Plaque reduces the flow of blood (traffic) and increases pressure in the artery (construction zone).

The total blockage of the artery may occur due to: a) the **buildup** of plaque, b) the formation of a blood clot on the plaque, or c) the plaque **rupturing** and causing a larger blood clot to form. The complete blockage of the artery is called an **occlusion**.

BLOOD FLOW

OCCLUSION

Why is HDL-cholesterol so useful?

HDL-cholesterol circulating through the bloodstream has many positive effects. HDL-cholesterol acts like a **scavenger** by helping to remove cholesterol from other lipoproteins in the bloodstream and from the artery wall. HDL-cholesterol takes the excess cholesterol back to the liver for its removal from the body.

HDL-CHOLESTEROL
REMOVING LDL-CHOLESTEROL
FROM THE BLOODSTREAM

What should my cholesterol levels be?

For individuals with two or more risk factors for cardiovascular disease, **LDL-cholesterol** should be **less than 130 mg/dL**. Risk factors include cigarette smoking, high blood pressure (more than 140/90 mm Hg) or use of antihypertensive medication, low **HDL-cholesterol** (less than 40 mg/dL), age (older than 45 for men and 55 for women), family history of premature heart disease, sedentary lifestyle and diabetes.

Other important values

For those individuals with coronary heart disease or diabetes, **LDL-cholesterol** should be **less than 100 mg/dL**. For individuals with two or more risk factors for cardiovascular disease, **LDL-cholesterol** should be **less than 130 mg/dL**.

Triglycerides should be **less than 200 mg/dL**.

HDL-cholesterol. This should be **greater than 40 mg/dL** for men and **more than 45 mg/dL** for women.

What are the first steps to reducing my risk factors for cardiovascular disease?

Without a doubt, quit smoking. Consult with your doctor about programs that are available to help you stop smoking. Two other steps that may help you to reduce your risk of cardiovascular disease are to **begin exercising** and to **modify your diet**. Here are some basic steps ...

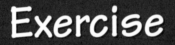

Currently, only 22% of adults in the United States exercise at a level that benefits their cardiovascular systems. What are some important considerations?

1) Type of exercise

2) Amount and regularity of exercise

3) Intensity of exercise

1. Type of exercise

Aerobic exercise

To meet your general fitness goals, the best type of exercise is **aerobic** exercise.

Aerobic exercise does not necessarily require special equipment or a health club membership. Aerobic exercises are those that require a lot of oxygen. These exercises include walking, jogging, cycling, swimming, cross-country skiing, or rowing.

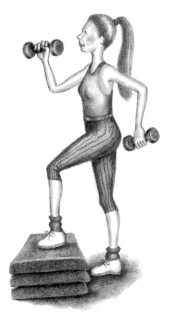

20-30 minutes a day, 5 days a week

2. Amount and regularity of exercise

The U.S. surgeon general recommends that healthy adults exercise 20 to 30 minutes, 5 days a week.

There are nearly 50 half hours in a 24-hour day. Exercising for 30 minutes daily requires **only about 2%** of your total day. Try to find 1, or 2, or 3 exercises you like to do. You'll enjoy the variety.

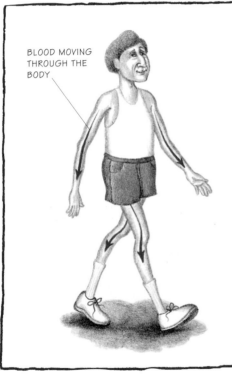

BLOOD MOVING THROUGH THE BODY

3. Intensity of exercise

Warm up

By walking or cycling slowly, you move the blood out to the working muscles. A warm-up should start slowly and last 5 to 10 minutes.

You cannot maintain "all out" exercise (100%) for very long. An example of an "all out" exercise is sprinting. Actually, you may only maintain a sprint for about 15 seconds.

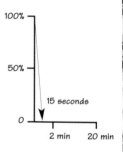

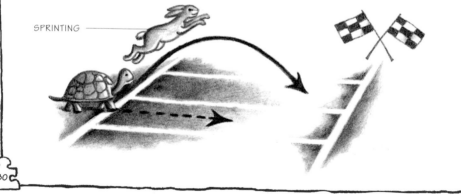

SPRINTING

If you slow the exercise down a bit, to about 90%, you may still only go for about 2 minutes!

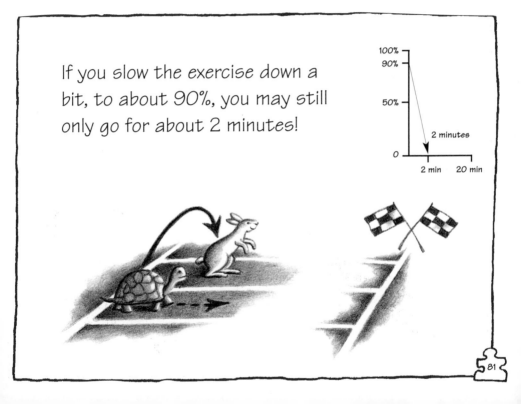

What if you slow your exercise down to 75% or even 50%? There is a **huge** difference. Now you may easily go more than 20 minutes.

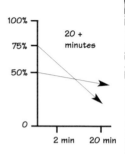

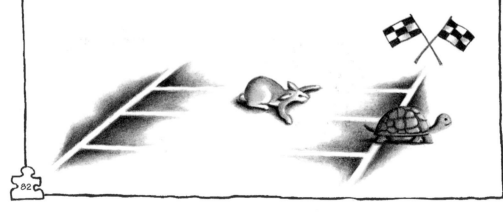

Simply —

By slowing down the pace, you may be able to exercise for a longer period of time.

Many exercise physiologists use the following generally accepted formula to determine the exercise target heart rate of a healthy individual. If you have a history of cardiovascular disease, or if you are just starting a program, **check with your doctor.** Your doctor is aware of the many factors that may need to be considered in modifying your exercise intensity.

Target heart rate example

Your age: 50

1. 220 minus your age:
2. Answer #1 minus your resting pulse:
3. Answer #2 times 0.5:
4. Answer #3 plus your resting pulse:
5. Answer #2 times 0.75:
6. Answer #5 plus your resting pulse:
7. **Target heart rate** equals range between values for #4 and #6:

Your resting pulse: 70

1. 220 - 50 = 170
2. 170 - 70 = 100
3. 100 x 0.5 = 50
4. 50 + 70 = 120
5. 100 x 0.75 = 75
6. 75 + 70 = 145
7. **120 to 145 beats per minute, or 12 to 14 beats for 6 seconds**

Now it's your turn

Here is how you determine the heart rate of an apparently healthy individual. Please consult with your doctor to make sure that this is an accurate target heart rate for your condition.

1. Measure your pulse (heart rate) for 60 seconds: _____
2. Take 220 and subtract your age: 220 - _____ = _____
3. Now take the answer in #2 and subtract your pulse: _____
4. Take the answer in #3 and multiply by 0.5: _____
5. Take the answer in #4 and add your pulse: _____
6. Take the answer in #3 and multiply by 0.75: _____
7. Take the answer in #6 and add your pulse: _____
8. Your target heart rate should range from the answer in
    #5 (_____) to the answer in #7 (_____).
9. Divide each answer in #8 by 10 to determine your
    pulse for 6 seconds: _____ to _____.

How hard and how often should I exercise?

When you are just starting out, try to exercise very comfortably. Here are 4 quick tips.

1) Try to exercise so that you are breathing noticeably but are **not** out of breath. Remember this simple rule: you should be able to carry on a conversation while you are exercising.

2) Sweating is a good thing. This means that your body is working hard enough and receiving the necessary stimulus for the muscles and the heart.

3) If you are not **fatigued** and are completely recovered from *exercising* on the previous day, then you should *exercise* **daily**.

4) Give yourself a **warm-up** before exercise (several minutes **of easy** walking) and a **cooldown** at the **end of** exercise (again, several minutes **of easy** walking). Ask an exercise specialist **for some** recommendations for stretching **after your** workout, and discuss the intensity of the exercise with your doctor.

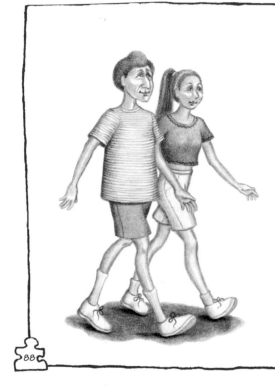

If you are just starting an exercise program, probably the simplest exercise to try is walking. It is fairly easy to do for 20 minutes. Check with your doctor for any additional input on your exercise program.

VERY, VERY important

Cool down. As important as the warm-up and the aerobic exercise are to improving your fitness, you must also include a cooldown as part of your exercise routine.

Your cooldown should be just like your warm-up. At the end of your exercise routine, give yourself 5 to 10 minutes of nice, easy walking. You also may want to include some mild stretching.

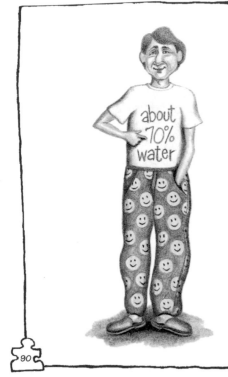

Another consideration — water

Water is needed for virtually every function of the body. The body is approximately 70% water.

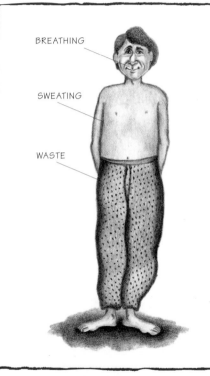

BREATHING

SWEATING

WASTE

During the course of the day, you lose water through sweating, breathing, and waste. Replacement of water (rehydration) is important — especially when participating in an exercise program.

A prudent recommendation is that you should drink 6 to 10 glasses of water per day. Sorry, caffeinated drinks and alcohol do not count. They are "diuretics," meaning that they actually may cause you to lose even more water.

In addition to exercise, the National Cholesterol Education Program recommends diet modification as another important factor in helping to lower your cholesterol.

Nutrition

As mentioned earlier, your body receives cholesterol two ways: the cholesterol made by your body in the liver and cholesterol you obtain from animal sources in the diet.

It is possible to lower your blood cholesterol by changing what you eat. Things that you can do to reduce your cholesterol vary by food group. Start by making changes in one area at a time.

Here's a brief review of the different food groups and how each can affect your blood cholesterol.

Fats

Not all fats are bad.

Monounsaturated fats are "good" fats. Examples of monounsaturated fats include olive and canola oils, peanut butter, and nuts.

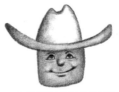

MONOUNSATURATED FAT

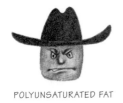

POLYUNSATURATED FAT

Polyunsaturated fats are "acceptable" fats. Examples of polyunsaturated fats include margarine made with corn or safflower oils and some nuts.

95

Saturated fats are the "bad" fats, particularly the **"trans" fats**. Saturated fats are usually solid at room temperature. Examples of saturated fats include lard, butter, and cream cheese. Examples of "trans" fats include partially hydrogenated vegetable oils found in many snack foods.

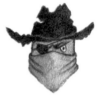

SATURATED FAT

It is difficult to eat a diet without saturated fat unless you are on a strict vegetarian diet. While we need fats in our diet, we also need to choose our foods wisely, especially meats, eggs, and dairy products.

People who have high cholesterol and are at risk for cardiovascular disease, and people who have had a cardiac event, should contact a dietitian about reducing their saturated fat intake and limiting their intake of alcohol, caffeine, and salt. The dietitian will also be able to review the amount of sugar you are eating — especially sugars found in "no fat" snack foods.

Meats

As mentioned, limit the amount of fatty meats, particularly those foods that are very high in saturated fats (bacon, sausage, and prime rib), to 1 or 2 servings per week. Cook meats using little or no fat, such as baking, broiling, grilling, stewing, or stir-frying without adding fat. Always trim off the obvious fat **before** cooking red meats and remove the skin before cooking chicken.

RED MEAT

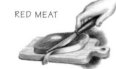

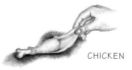

CHICKEN

Eggs

It used to be thought that these were the main culprits of elevated cholesterol. This may not be true. However, if you have elevated cholesterol or a history of heart disease, you should limit egg yolks to no more than 3 or 4 per week. Egg whites or "egg substitutes" have no cholesterol and do not need to be limited.

EGGS

Dairy products

Switch from whole milk to 2% and then to 1% or even skim milk. Use low-fat cheeses, yogurt, and sour cream. For a healthier dessert, look for low-fat ice cream or sherbet.

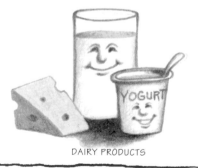

DAIRY PRODUCTS

Whole grains, fruits, and vegetables

Another thing you can do to help improve your overall diet is to eat a variety of healthier foods. The American Heart Association recommends that you try to increase the number of servings of foods that are high in whole grains, such as breads and cereals, and try to have at least **5 servings** of fruits and vegetables every day.

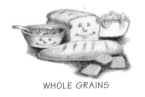

WHOLE GRAINS

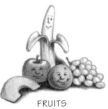

FRUITS

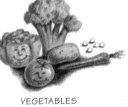

VEGETABLES

What else can be done to reduce your chances of developing heart disease?

Despite the changes you may make in your diet and exercise routine, it may still be necessary for you to consider medication. Your doctor will closely monitor your progress with the dietitian. Then you and your doctor will be able to decide on the type of medical therapy that is best for you.

Medications, Angioplasty, and Bypass Surgery

Treating blocked arteries

An artery that is completely blocked has no blood flowing through it. If the heart muscle does not receive blood, then it does not receive nutrients and oxygen. When the heart does not receive oxygen, it experiences **ischemia**. This may result in **heart pain** (angina) or a **heart attack**. **Ischemia**, if prolonged and severe enough, may cause a portion of the heart muscle to die (heart attack).

BLOCKAGE

LACK OF
BLOOD FLOW

What are some symptoms of a possible heart attack?

- **Angina**, or heart pain, usually felt as a pressure, ache, tightness, squeezing, or **burning sensation** under the breastbone and often extending to the neck, jaw, shoulders, or down the arm (most frequently the left arm)
- **Nausea**
- **Shortness of breath** and/or **sweating**

Interestingly, **diabetic patients** do not "feel" angina in the same way and are more than twice as likely as nondiabetics to have a "silent" or unrecognized heart attack.

Quite often, people who are having a heart attack say they feel like "an elephant is standing on my chest."

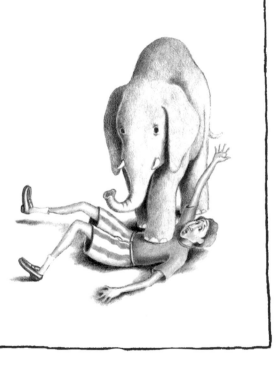

Statins

Several years ago, a class of medications was introduced to help reduce the amount of cholesterol in the bloodstream.

This class of medications is collectively known as **Statins**. Studies have shown that this group of medications is very effective for most people in helping to **reduce** their total cholesterol, LDL-cholesterol, and triglycerides and — in some instances — **increase** the HDL-cholesterol.

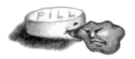 This is particularly important for individuals who have already been diagnosed with coronary heart disease or who have already had a cardiac event.

Patients who are not candidates for therapy with Statins include those individuals who have liver damage or have allergies to these medications. As with all medications, be sure you consult with your doctor about the recommended dosage.

Thrombolytics

Most often, a heart attack is caused by a **blood clot** (thrombus) at a site of **atherosclerotic plaque disruption** within the coronary artery. Blood clots can completely block blood flow in the artery and cause a heart attack. If a person gets to a hospital emergency room, usually within 30 minutes of the onset of chest pain, a class of medications called **thrombolytics** may be used to dissolve these clots and restore coronary blood flow. The restoration of blood flow to the heart muscle can save heart muscle and reduce the chance of dying.

Thrombolytics are most beneficial if given soon after the onset of heart attack symptoms.

Certain individuals may not be candidates to receive thrombolytics, including those who have had a recent stroke, surgery, or trauma that would increase the risk of serious bleeding. Likewise, individuals with bleeding peptic ulcers, very high blood pressure, or very advanced age may be at increased risk with thrombolytic therapy. An alternative treatment to thrombolytic therapy for a heart attack is **coronary angioplasty**.

Angioplasty

Angioplasty is a procedure by which the cardiologist inserts a balloon catheter over a thin wire across a blockage of a coronary artery.

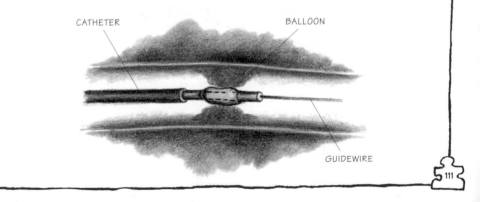

CATHETER

BALLOON

GUIDEWIRE

The balloon is inflated to compress the plaque.
This is repeated as necessary by the cardiologist.

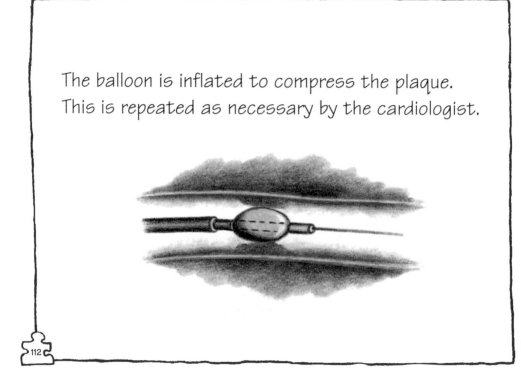

Inflating the catheter compresses and breaks apart the plaque. This allows more room for the blood to flow.

The balloon catheter also stretches the elastic wall of the artery. Small tears occur on the inside of the artery wall and slightly injure the artery wall as a result of balloon catheter inflation.

BLOOD FLOW

Unfortunately, these balloon catheter injuries expose substances from inside the atherosclerotic plaque and the artery wall that promote formation of blood clots.

Complications of this procedure may include a heart attack, repeat angioplasty, the need for emergency coronary bypass surgery, and even death.

Stents

In certain instances, the cardiologist may decide to insert a **stent** inside the coronary artery. The stent, usually made of stainless steel, functions as a scaffold to hold open the inside of the coronary artery.

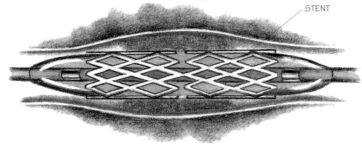

STENT

Stents are usually put in place using a balloon angioplasty catheter. Stents can reduce the incidence of both short- and long-term coronary artery reocclusion. Stents can seal and "tack up" tissue flaps within the artery that are created when a balloon catheter injures the artery. Unfortunately, stents do not eliminate clot formation or the occurrence of heart attack following the procedure.

Bypass surgery

Bypass surgery is a cardiovascular procedure designed to correct blood flow to the heart that angioplasty cannot correct. The cardiovascular surgeon uses a piece of artery and/or vein to reroute blood around the blockage.

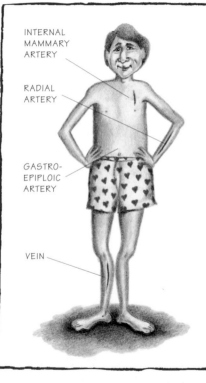

INTERNAL
MAMMARY
ARTERY

RADIAL
ARTERY

GASTRO-
EPIPLOIC
ARTERY

VEIN

The surgeon may use a vein
from the leg, and/or the
internal mammary artery
found in the chest, and/or
the gastroepiploic artery
of the stomach, and/or
the radial artery of the
forearm.

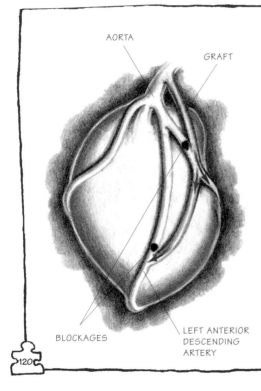

AORTA

GRAFT

BLOCKAGES

LEFT ANTERIOR DESCENDING ARTERY

The vein is attached to the aorta. The supply of blood is then rerouted around the blockage. One piece of vein may be used for multiple bypasses. The number of blockages where blood has been rerouted — not the number of veins used — determines the number of bypasses.

If the internal mammary artery is used, the artery originates from a branch off the aorta and is attached directly below the blockage.

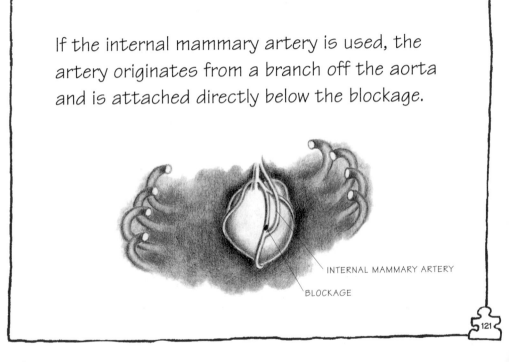

INTERNAL MAMMARY ARTERY

BLOCKAGE

What about 'after care' from a heart attack, bypass surgery, or angioplasty?

Your doctor will manage your care very closely. Generally, the cardiologist may recommend that you:

- quit smoking
- take a beta blocker drug (after a heart attack)
- lower your LDL-cholesterol below 100 mg/dL
- take a daily enteric-coated aspirin (81 mg or greater) unless you have other medical complications
- follow a "heart-healthy diet" and begin a basic exercise program, mainly walking. Always follow your doctor's recommendations.

Questions

Here are some questions that you may want to take with you the next time you go to see your doctor.

What are my medications? How does each of them help me?

Answer

_____

_____

_____

_____

_____

_____

_____

125

List the total cholesterol (TC), LDL-cholesterol (LDL), HDL-cholesterol (HDL), and triglycerides (Trig) readings for each visit to your doctor.

Date	TC	LDL	HDL	Trig

Based on my weight, blood pressure, and blood cholesterol level, should I talk to someone about changing my diet?

Yes   No

Contact your local hospital for the name of a registered dietitian.

Dietitian _____

Address _____

_____

Phone _____

Do I have any exercise limitations of which I should be aware? What are they?

Answer _____

_____

Should I have a treadmill test before I start to exercise? What is my target heart rate?

Answer _____

_____

128

Are there any concerns that I should be aware of before having/resuming sexual activity?

Answer _____

_____

_____

_____

And now some
heartfelt thoughts ...

For more than 50% of the individuals who have cardiovascular disease, the first sign is a **fatal heart attack**. It has been mentioned throughout the book, but the importance of seeing your doctor and having a complete physical exam cannot be stressed enough. If necessary, sit down with a dietitian and review your current eating pattern. Then, if your doctor agrees, get moving. Start a simple exercise program — mainly walking. There are no guarantees you will reduce your risk of having a cardiac event, but at least you will be taking an aggressive approach to improving your health.

Bibliography

American College of Sports Medicine position stand. "The Recommended Quality and Quantity of Exercise for Developing and Maintaining Cardiorespiratory and Muscular Fitness in Healthy Adults." *Medicine and Science in Sports and Exercise* April 1990.

Angell, M. "Caring for women's health – what is the problem?" *New England Journal of Medicine* 1993: 271.

Burke, A.P., and A. Farb, G.T. Malcom, Y. Liang, J. Smialek, R. Virmani. "Coronary Risk Factors and Plaque Morphology in Men with Coronary Disease Who Died Suddenly." *New England Journal of Medicine* 1 May 1997: 1276-1282.

Cogswell, M.E. "Nicotine Withdrawal Symptoms." *North Carolina Medical Journal* 1 Jan. 1995: 40-45.

Collins, R., and R. Peto, C. Baigent, P. Sleight. "Aspirin, Heparin, and Fibrinolytic Therapy in Suspected Acute Myocardial Infarction." *New England Journal of Medicine* 20 March 1997: 847-860.

Da Costa, F.D., et al. "Myocardial Revascularization with the Radial Artery: A Clinical and Angiographic Study." *Annals of Thoracic Surgery* Aug. 1996: 475-480.

Eckel, R.H. "Obesity in Heart Disease." *Circulation* 1997: 3248-3250.

Executive Summary of the Third Report of the National Cholesterol Education Program (NCEP) Expert Panel on Detection, Evaluation, and Treatment of High Blood Cholesterol in Adults (Adult Treatment Panel III). JAMA, May 16, 2001, Vol. 285, No. 19: 2486-2497.

Friedman, G.D., and A.L. Klatsky. "Is Alcohol Good for Your Health?" *New England Journal of Medicine* 16 Dec. 1993: 1882-1883.

Gellar, A. "Common Addictions." *Clinical Symposia*. Ciba-Geigy Corporation 1996.

Grossman, E., and F.H. Messerli. "Diabetic and Hypertensive Heart Disease." *Annals of Internal Medicine* 15 Aug. 1996: 304-310.

Henningfield, J.D., and R.M. Keenan. "The Anatomy of Nicotine Addiction." *Health Values* March/April 1993: 12-19.

Joint National Committee. The Fifth Report of the Joint National Committee on Detection, Evaluation, and Treatment of High Blood Pressure. Bethesda (MD): National Institutes of Health, National Heart, Lung, and Blood Institute; 1993. NIH publication No. 93-1008.

Kannel, W.B., and R.B. D'Agostino, J.L. Cobb. "Effects of Weight on Cardiovascular Disease." *American Journal of Clinical Nutrition* March 1996: 419S-422S.

Katzel, L.I., et al. "Effects of an American Heart Association step I diet and weight loss on lipoprotein lipid levels in obese men with silent myocardial ischemia and reduced highdensity lipoprotein cholesterol." Metabolism: Clinical & Experimental. March 1995: 307-314.

Kenney, W.L. et al. *American College of Sports Medicine Guidelines for Exercise Testing and Prescription.* 5th ed. Media, Pa.: Williams & Wilkins, 1995.

Margolis, S., and P.J. Goldschmidt-Clermont. *The Johns-Hopkins White Papers.* Baltimore: The Johns-Hopkins Medical Institutions, 1996.

McCarron, D.A., and M.E. Reusser. "Body Weight and Blood Pressure Regulation." *American Journal of Clinical Nutrition* March 1996: 423S-425S.

Meeker, M.H., and J.C. Rothrock. *Alexander's Care of the Patient in Surgery,* 10th ed. St. Louis: Mosby, 1995.

Peterson, J.A., and C.X. Bryant. *The Fitness Handbook;* 2nd ed. St. Louis: Wellness Bookshelf, 1995.

Ryan, T.J., and J.L. Anderson, E.M. Autman, et al. "ACC/AHA Guidelines for the Management of Patients with Acute Myocardial Infarction: A Report of the American College of Cardiology/American Heart Association Task Force on Practice Guidelines (Committee on Management of Acute Myocardial Infarction)." *Journal of the American College of Cardiology* 1 Nov. 1996: 1328-1428.

St. Jeor, S.T., and K.D. Brownell, R.L. Atkinson, C. Bouchard, et al. "Obesity Workshop III." *Circulation* 1996: 1391-1396.

Schlant, R.C., and R.W. Alexander. *The Heart*, 8th ed. New York: McGraw-Hill, 1994.

Superko, H.R. "The Most Common Cause of Coronary Heart Disease can be Successfully Treated by the Least Expensive Therapy — Exercise." *Certified News* 1998: 1-5.

United States Surgeon General. Department of Health and Human Services. *The Health Consequences of Smoking. Nicotine Addiction.* Washington, D.C.: U.S. Department of Health and Human Services, 1988.

United States Surgeon General on his priorities at http://www.osophs.dhhs.gov/myjob/priorities.htm accessed November 1999.

Voors, A.A., et al. "Smoking and Cardiac Events After Venous Coronary Bypass Surgery." *Circulation* Jan. 1, 1995: 42-47.

Voutilainen, S., et al. "Angiographic 5-Year Follow-up Study of Right Gastroepiploic Artery Grafts." *Annals of Thoracic Surgery* Aug. 1996: 501-505.

White H.D., and J.J. Van de Werf. "Thrombolysis for Acute Myocardial Infarction." *Circulation* 28 April 1998: 1632-1646.

Zelasko, C.J. "Exercise for Weight Loss: What are the Facts?" *Journal of the American Dietetic Association* Dec. 1995: 973-1031.

Notes

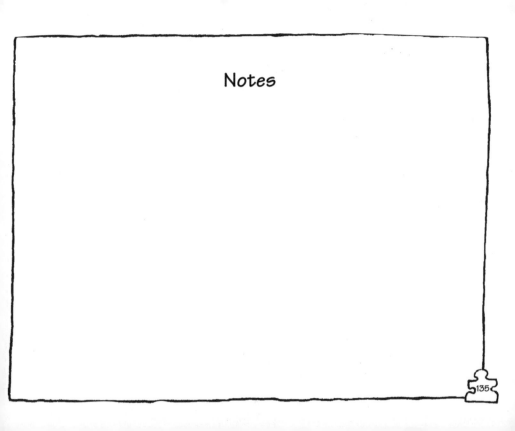

About the Authors

Dean J. Kereiakes, MD, FACC, is one of the nation's preeminent cardiologists. Dr. Kereiakes is President of the Ohio Heart Health Center, Medical Director of the Carl and Edyth Lindner Center for Clinical Cardiovascular Research, Professor of Clinical Medicine at the University of Cincinnati, and Professor of Medicine at The Ohio State University. He frequently lectures worldwide and has published hundreds of articles and papers. Dr. Kereiakes lives in Cincinnati, Ohio.

Douglas Wetherill, MS, is Supervisor of Disease Management at a large Midwest manufacturing company. He lives in Cincinnati, Ohio.

For additional copies of *High Cholesterol: What You Should Know*™,
please contact your local bookseller or call (800) 216-2522

For institutional quantities, contact our Special Sales Department at
rsime@blacksci.com or call (800) 759-6102

Other titles in the series *Your Health: What You Should Know*™:

Congestive Heart Failure: What You Should Know™
Diabetes: What You Should Know™
Heart Disease: What You Should Know™
Women's Health Over 40: What You Should Know™
Women's Health Under 40: What You Should Know™

DISCARDED
New Hanover County Public Library

136

D0682970

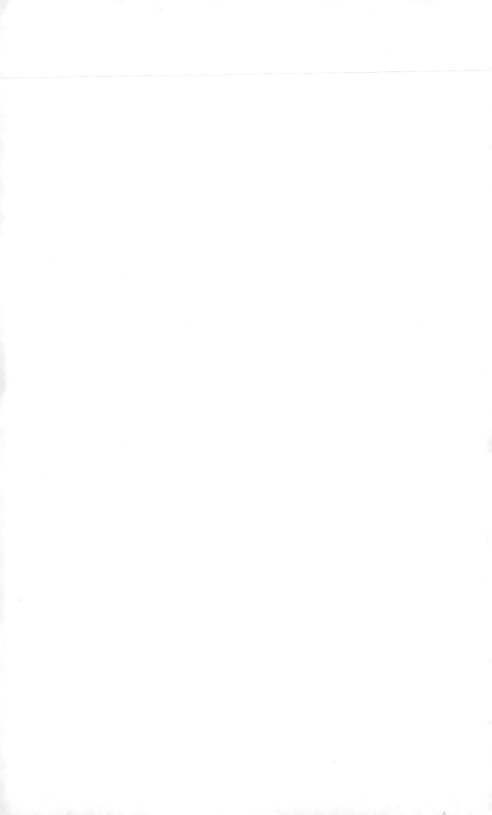

SO IT WAS

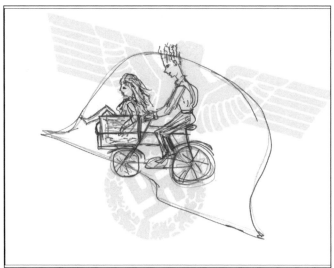

Stephanie and me off to see the Tiger

SO IT WAS

One man's recollections
of the
German Occupation
of Jersey
from boyhood to manhood
1940 to 1945

Richard Weithley

CHANNEL ISLAND PUBLISHING

First published in 2001.
Revised and reprinted
in 2003, 2005 & 2007 by
Channel Island Publishing
Unit 3b, Barette Commercial Centre
La Route du Mont Mado
St John, Jersey JE3 4DS

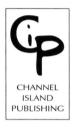

CHANNEL
ISLAND
PUBLISHING

We acknowledge with thanks permission to
reproduce photographs supplied by
Société Jersiaise Photographic Archive, Jersey

© Richard Weithley
All rights reserved. No part of this publication may be reproduced,
stored in a retrieval system or transmitted in any form or by any means
without the prior written permission of the publisher.

Printed by The Cromwell Press, Trowbridge, Wiltshire

ISBN 0 9525659 6 X

Dedicated to my Mother
Mona Agnes Williams
(née Le Gallais)

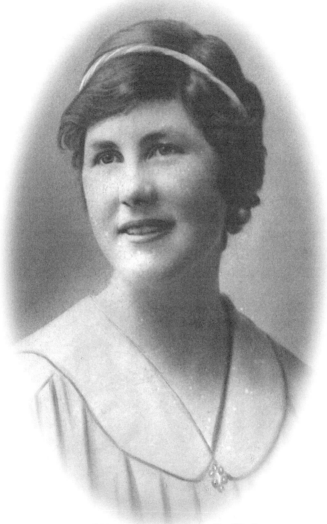

Mona Agnes Le Gallais
Circa 1920

"....and as they ran they looked behind and snatched a fearful joy "

CONTENTS

Acknowledgments

The publisher would like to thank the following for their kind assistance in the production of this publication.

Simon Watkins	Cover design
Alan Lagadu	Cover Photography
John Quemard	Production co-ordinator
Robert Daly	Cover Model
Hannah Le Couilliard	Cover Model
Island Fortress	Occupation Bike
Michel Garcia	Artist Impressions
Ruth Curzon	Typing

CHAPTER 1

SO IT WAS

This story starts in June 1940 and will end in May 1945. Its content and *raison d'etre* concern the German Occupation of Jersey during that period. It will tell, or attempt to tell, with all due truthfulness and reasonable modesty, of some deprivation, many happy times, capture and escape, luck and larceny, love, lunacy, sabotage, a shipwreck, fearful joy and much else.

The Germans bombed Jersey on 28th June, 1940. It was early evening and I was standing in gardens near my family's home, Sunnyside, Marrett Road, at Havre des Pas on the outskirts of St Helier. Looking across towards Fort Regent, I could see the German bombers circling the town and docks area of St Helier.

As I watched, the bomb hatches opened and strings of bombs could clearly be seen until they disappeared behind Fort Regent. Explosions followed and then smoke rising above the Fort. There were only three or four bombers and the air raid was of short duration. I was later given to understand that the Germans were merely testing the Island's defences, if any. There were none and the *Luftwaffe* had their little fun whilst many Jerseymen died in earnest.

Local people stood in excited groups in the streets in animated conversation. They had little, if any, knowledge of bombs or wars. Certainly I had none. As a boy of fourteen, I had little to say but with ears big enough to listen to the chatter. Would the Germans come to Jersey? The consensus of opinion was that they would not. Jersey had no troops and was of no importance, so why would they bother themselves.

A little old grey haired man said that those swine would come and we had all better go home as they may return with more bombs at any minute. I took him at his word and at home I suffered more from an anxious mother and father than I had from the *Luftwaffe*.

1

The town was strangely quiet on the Saturday and Sunday. People did their shopping, gossiped but fear and trepidation was abroad. Some, with both worldly experience and money, had already started heavy purchasing of canned food and luxuries.

On the Monday following the air raid, I was able to see some of the damage caused as I was, at that time, employed by a Mr Foster at his radio shop at the top of Hill Street opposite Snow Hill Bus Station in St Helier. Mr Foster, on that Air Raid Friday, was in the bar of the Yacht Hotel near the Weighbridge having his after work drink. His car, among a row of others, had been parked in Mulcaster Street. Either incendiary bombs or tracer bullets had hit this row of cars and they caught fire. Mr Foster and I went to look at the damage and he made arrangements to have his car, a complete wreck, towed to a garage he owned in Union Street.

The Germans arrived on the 1st of July, 1940 and soon after were much in evidence in the streets. These were victorious troops, well attired in their various uniforms, marching, bands playing, strutting and singing. I particularly remember a very German marching song, although the tune is better remembered than the words. It was something like: 'Hi he hi ho, hi ho, hi he hi ho, hi he, hi ho, hi hah hah hah...'

This was show-off, the marching, singing troops were going nowhere. Just up and down like the Grand Old Duke of York's men.

Swastikas were everywhere, as were pictures of Hitler, very occasionally improved by the addition of glasses and beard, the work of some intrepid local artists.

Other causes for amusement were not lacking. One such was the Union Jack logo mounted on the bonnet of a certain make of a british cars, a Standard, commandeered by the Germans for use by officers. It was many weeks before they were removed from their frames. In the mind's eye, the empty frame still contained the Union Jack.

The German troops and their sometimes weird goings on, such as the goosestep, *Heil Hitlers*, crashing of their boot heels with upraised arm salute, were a novelty and as a nine day wonder they lasted perhaps a month or two. It is important to understand that two very different societies developed over the Occupation years: the Germans and us. We learned to ignore them unless, as from time to time, their stupidity and barbarism were forced on us, causing discomfort and often pain.

It is again of some importance to know that owing to the evacuation to Britain of many thousands of Jersey people in early 1940 and immigration after the war, the local population of Jersey during the Occupation would have been twenty-five percent of the present day numbers. In St Helier almost all were known, one to the other.

Further, Jersey was largely self supporting. Farms were active working units with cows, pigs and poultry. Cider apple trees were common and barrels of cider were to be found in the farmers' barns. In late spring when the early potatoes were harvested, the fields were immediately planted with many different types of vegetables. We might have fared reasonably well if our rapacious visitors had left us alone.

My first direct encounters with German troops occurred at my work at Foster's Radio Shop. I had left school, St.Luke's near Georgetown, at the age of fourteen, my fourteenth birthday being in April, 1940. I had started at Fosters in May as assistant and delivery boy. My job was mainly recharging customers' wet batteries, town deliveries and serving in the shop when the shop manager or sales girl were at lunch or away on some other business. If anyone wished to buy anything, I rang a bell for Mr Foster up in the repair room.

The work of battery charging took place twice each week. These were wet batteries for radios. This was a simple job of placing them on the charging table, topping them up, wiring them together, positive and negatives in one continuous line and switching on the charger. They stayed on charge overnight. The charging room was in the basement, the whole ground floor area was the shop. Offices were on the first floor and the repair facility at second floor level where Mr Foster spent most of his working time.

From time to time during my work in the shop German soldiers came in. They seldom bought anything but just looked around and left. We did not sell records but we sold record players, needles, record cleaners and such odds and ends. Three or four times I was caught by a sly joke of the Germans. They would come in and ask for the record: 'We're going to hang out the washing on the Siegfried Line, have you any dirty washing, mother dear?' This was a recording made by Flanagan and Allen in early 1940. This request was always accompanied by smirks and great glee. Other than to say no, that we did not sell records, there was little to be done. They were crowing and triumphant and some humiliation on our part was suffered. My only response, silent, was 'Go home Adolf.' Mr Foster was in the shop on one such occasion and the same enquiry was made to him. His reply: 'The record is presently out of print but would be reprinted when the time is right.'

My real mishap came when, one fine day in August, I was on duty in the shop during the lunch period. I was alone in the shop when two soldiers came in. They were typical, tall, blond, in their mid twenties, healthy and assured, with their own German soldiers smell, a combination of gun oil, leather, cologne and a dash of sweat. In later years the cologne would be replaced by many more dashes of sweat.

Entering the shop, one followed the display shelves to the right or left, which followed the walls of the shop until left and right met in the back section of the shop. There were four display tables in the centre areas and on one was a blue, soft leather covered 'Pye' portable radio - not much bigger than a ladies vanity case. I stood and watched them until the one to the left called me over to question me on the price of a particular radio, then moved on asking questions on other radios. He thanked me and left the shop, his friend had gone before him and so, I discovered, had the Pye.

I rang the shop bell, which sounded upstairs, for assistance and Mr Foster came down. The story was explained and he called the police. A local policeman soon arrived and the story again repeated. Off he went. He must have explained it all to his superior as within an hour a local police officer and a German officer appeared. All was once more described.

'There must be some mistake' said the German officer. 'Soldiers of the Third Reich do not steal.'

'They do and have' was my insistent reply.

A crazy series of events followed. He left the shop and returned in ten minutes with two soldiers very similar in appearance to my description. 'Are these the men?'

'No!'

He repeated this exercise four times, with, of course, no result. There were hundreds of similar German soldiers on the streets of St Helier at that time. I explained that they all looked the same to me and unless he could find two with a blue Pye, a portable radio set, his efforts were in vain. He finally left, German honour satisfied.

Mr Foster never regained his radio and I received a telling off with threats to deduct the cost from my wages which, at three shillings and sixpence a week, would have seen me without wages for thirty weeks, stony broke amid the enemy.

Mr Foster never made good his threat but I was no longer allowed to keep shop. My duties were now entirely devoted to battery charging and deliveries. In a very short time, the latter became my main occupation as the delivery van, due to shortages of petrol, was no longer allowed to be used and the delivery bike the only means of transport. The stock of radios was soon exhausted and deliveries consisted of batteries and radios for repair and repaired.

I was now to enter Arcadia and reside there for a lovely but too short time. My deliveries covered the whole Island but I was more often in Rozel than elsewhere. Mr Foster lived in a house overlooking the sea at the top of Rozel on the St Martin side. This house is now a restaurant called Frère de Mer.

At least three times each week something or other had to be taken to or from the house and it was on one of my many trips that I met Stephanie. Stephanie lived in St Martin quite close to the church. She lived with two aunts as her mother and father were not living together and she often walked to Rozel Manor where her mother was employed. In my rides to Mr Foster's house I had sometimes passed her and one fine September afternoon I caught up with her on La Grande Route de Rozel.

In her walk she had just reached the bottom of the hill where a stream runs under the road and a lodge nestled among the trees of a wood bordering the road. From here, the road immediately climbed toward the junction with the Rue des Alleurs and Rozel Manor a little further on toward Rozel. As the rise was steep, it was convenient to dismount and push the bike and much more convenient to dismount near Stephanie and start a conversation. We chatted happily and when we reached the top of the hill I continued walking with her until we reached the gates of Rozel Manor.

Thereafter we met two or three times a week - which were to become three or four and Saturdays added. Stephanie increased her visits to her mother or just went for a walk. My delivery bike had a large container frame achieved by the front wheel being one quarter the size of the rear. I always had a large cardboard box, reinforced with a plywood sheet at the base of the box, placed within the metal container frame. After meeting Stephanie I had a piece of lino and carpet cut to the size of the cardboard box. Stephanie and I would go for rides with Stephanie sitting in the box. The lino and carpet were to protect her from any acid that may have spilled from the batteries. If I had items still in the box, these were removed, hidden under bushes to be collected and delivered later. I once forgot a radio and it stayed under the bushes all night. I collected it early next morning, safe and sound, but rather damp. Its owner accepted my excuses for being late and also my request that it be placed before the fire before connection to the electric mains. It was such a damp morning! It was a sturdy radio: it crackled for a while when first switched on, but it did not blow up. When I told this story to Stephanie, she squeezed my hand and said that I was very clever! Insofar as she giggled throughout the rest of our visit, she must have thought me a scallywag, albeit a clever one.

We went blackberrying, to the seashore, hid in barns and under trees when it was wet and talked and talked and talked. She was altogether beautiful. Long fair hair, bright blue eyes, slim of figure, animated and with a bright, enquiring intelligence. Her steady regard for me increased my own confidence and volubility. Stephanie, my love, my dove, my only one.

It was not always easy to meet Stephanie, as deliveries would sometimes take me to the west of the Island but I almost always made it and the times that she waited in vain, if heartbreaking, were few. On such occasions she told me with her angelic smile, that she did not mind - she knew that she would see me the next day.

My efforts to meet with Stephanie became ingenious and no General ever planned the logistics of operations as well as I did. I became the demon delivery boy, Hermes, riding at breakneck speed through the parishes, waving to passers by, the 3.50pm express heading for the North. I lost weight for I rode in excess of twenty miles on most days, but I was fit and filled with joy. Mrs Le Brun's bakery at First Tower, Colonel Swan's radio at Beaumont, up St Peter's Valley for Vautier and Kevin's batteries. Through St Mary, past the road to St.Lawrence where I should have turned off for deliveries for Mrs Vibert and Mr Jack, I would return there after seeing Stephanie. On through Trinity, through the Rue des Alleure, down the hill to find Stephanie leaning against the railings in the dip of the hills near the lodge among the trees where the bluebells grew in the Spring. Triumph! Smiles and grins, life was regained and all was right in our small world. We sometimes had little more than half an hour and I would walk Stephanie home in the dark then go on to St Lawrence to finish my deliveries.

Such late rides were beautiful on moonlight nights, birds calling, the tips of branches edged with silver. There were very few people about and I could dream and sing in happy solitude. Songs remain in the memory of happy times and I remember riding along in tree shadowed lanes singing: 'I'm only a wandering vagabond, so good night pretty maiden good night. I'm bound for the hills and the valleys beyond, so good night pretty maiden good night.' Stephanie was the prettiest of maidens.

I mentioned Colonel Swan earlier. He was a retired Indian Army man who lived at Beaumont on the back road between the cannon and Sandybrook. He was a sweet old man, tall, lanky and very thin, white hair but little of it. His face was exceedingly lined but he had kept his Indian tan. He was the oldest man I knew at that time...but only in years. He was the youngest old man I have ever known, he was my friend.

He was seldom still, at least when I was with him. He walked up and down his drawing room, waving and gesticulating and bade me be a good lad. He had pictures of himself in India, in uniform and at one time he had worn a beard. When I asked why he had shaved it off he said that bald men should not wear beards as other people always wanted to turn their heads upside down!

In the days of my sadness he tried his best to comfort me; mainly by letting me see his tiger as often as I wished. Colonel Swan's radio was always in for repair. I must have collected it and delivered it back repaired once every two weeks. It was said that it always needed repair because he beat it up when the news was bad.

On the floor of his sitting room he had the most beautiful tiger skin complete with paws, tail and head. It had cruel looking teeth and green eyes which I think were some type of semi-precious stones. They were very well chosen, for they had orange flecks and black pupils. I was fascinated to the extent that I would lie on the floor inches from the tiger's head and imagine meeting it in the Indian jungle. I often stayed there for half an hour or more and he would tell me stories of India, of the Moguls and Rajas, of the heat that shrivelled your bones, monsoon rains that choked you. Where a Man was a Man! 'Always be a Pukka Sahib my boy' he often repeated.

When he saw that I had to go, he would yell to his housekeeper, 'Iso, Iso, don't keep my guest waiting, he wants his bread and butter.' I think that her name was Isobel, a large plump lady, as kind and as sweet as her master. She brought me a thick slice of bread smothered in butter. Although he grumbled at her for keeping his guest waiting, she must have prepared the bread and butter awaiting his call. She told him that she took more care of this poor boy than he did - 'so be quiet!' This exchange was common and caused no concern. He always called me 'lad' and she called me 'my poor boy.'

Much later when radio sets were not allowed and I had learned to make crystal sets, I took one to Colonel Swan as a gift but he was no longer there. Other people now lived in the house and informed me that he had died and in my distress, I solicited no further information. I threw the crystal set in the brook at Sandybrook, for it belonged to Colonel Swan. The tiger had gone and so had he.

Stephanie and I remained incapable of being separated. We continued our rides, Stephanie sitting in the cardboard box facing forward, her long fair hair blowing in the wind and caressing my finger tips on the bike's handlebars. I purposely rode with my hands half way along the handlebars to ensure contact with her hair. We forgot Germans and much else. We sometimes met with marching troops, who called and waved. Lorries passed and horns were blown but we paid little attention.

The weather grew cold and wet, so we often went to a barn we had discovered on the Rue des Alleurs. It had no door and was holed and dirty but we huddled together, partly on and under an old overcoat of my father's which I carried with me if I was to meet with Stephanie. Of course, I told her of Colonel Swan and some of my other customers. She was particularly interested in the tiger and wished that she could see it. This could have been arranged but she was circumscribed by her aunts who otherwise treated her very well. Such work as they gave to her was mainly in the mornings helping about the house.

She was happy but sometimes wistful. 'Have no fear, dear Stephanie' I said. 'I shall take you to see the tiger. One day we shall go to India and see real tigers, even if our bones shrivel in the heat and we half drown in waterfalls of rain. I shall be a Pukka Sahib and you will be my Indian Princess.'

She shuddered when the heat shrivelled our bones and huddled closer. Both her hands clasped mine when we were drowned by the rain and she jumped up in delight at becoming an Indian Princess.

One late afternoon, darkness had fallen and I was taking Stephanie home when we were caught in a heavy shower of rain. We were in the dip of the hill near the lodge. We sheltered in the porch of the lodge and we kissed for the first and only time. We were both fourteen years of age. To talk, to hold hands, laugh and plan the impossible was the whole of life for me. The kiss, cold lips barely touching, was a pledge of trust and love. The rain had stopped and I took Stephanie home to her aunt's house. I never saw her again.

She was not there two days later where we had planned to meet, nor in the days that followed. I rode my bike between the church and the manor over and over again in fearful hope but she never came. Her aunts must have noticed me, for on one of my lonely vigils outside her aunts' house, the door of the house opened and a lady waved to me and

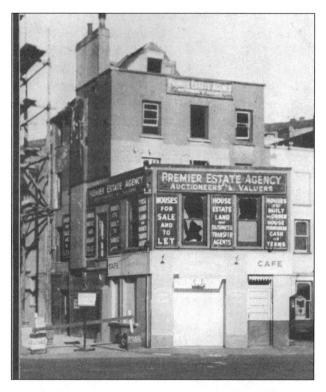

Bomb damage and machine gun bullet marks at 6.45pm on the 28th of June, 1940, in St Helier.

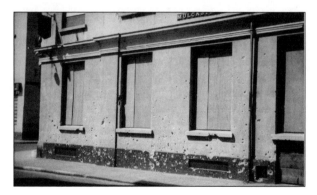

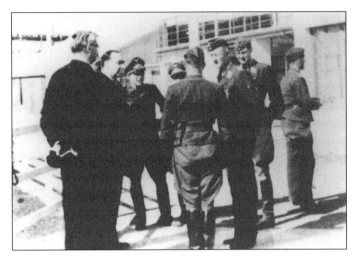

The first Germans arrive at Jersey Airport.

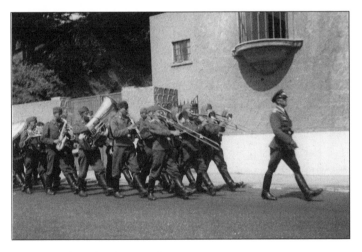

Military bands play in the streets.
Hi He Hi Ho Hi Ho.

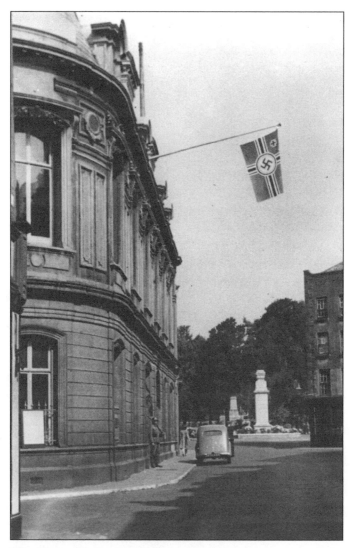

The Town Hall in St Helier.
Soon all public buildings are taken over.

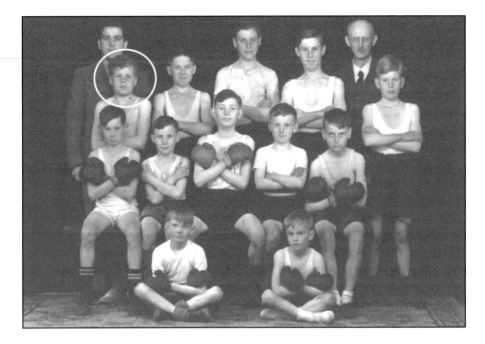

St Luke's School, 1939.

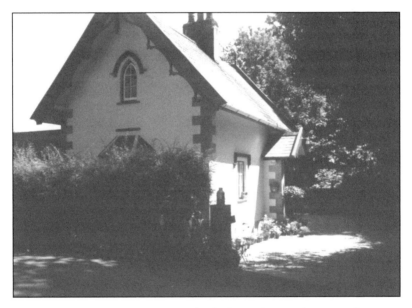

The Lodge in the dip in the hill on the road to Rozel.

called me to come in. They knew that I was the boy who had often been seen with Stephanie and asked if I was looking for her. I nodded but did not speak for I was distressed and embarrassed.

'Stephanie has left us,' said one of the aunts. 'Her mother has gone back to her husband. She and Stephanie now live in St Mary.' The aunts either did not know or did not wish to tell me, for when I asked 'Where in St Mary?' They said that they did not know. In pain, I started for the door but they stopped me, said that I must be cold and tired and must take a hot drink and eat a piece of cake. They sat me down and left to fetch the drink and cake. I was very near to tears and sat silently looking down at the floor, fiercely reminding myself that Pukka Sahibs do not cry. One of the aunts returned with the food and drink. They had told me that their names were Miss Jessica and Miss Vera.

I sipped the milk but was undone by my first bite of the cake. Tears started to fall and I could only sit there, unable to chew and wishing to hide away. They looked at each other then left the room. I swallowed the mouthful of cake as best I could and stuffed the rest in my pocket. I tried to drink the milk but left half of it. When they returned a few minutes later I was reasonably composed and, as I walked to the door, they handed me a bag of vegetables, saying that living in the town my mother would be pleased to have fresh vegetables. They asked me to call again soon. I did call but there was no news of Stephanie.

I called on them twice more, still hoping for news of Stephanie but received none. They always gave me bags of vegetables and, as they may have thought that I called only for that reason, I did not call again.

I rode my bike throughout St Mary for weeks afterwards but never saw Stephanie. Whenever I rode past the lodge amid the trees in the dip of the hill on my way to Rozel, a sweet nostalgia filled me with sadness.

So it was for Stephanie and me.

CHAPTER 2
MR DALES BOOT SHOP

M r Foster's stock of radio sets were entirely exhausted by November 1940. The business from then on was to rely entirely on repairs and charging of batteries. The staff was reduced to the manager and myself. Mr Foster came in to work by bicycle two or three times a week, or depending upon the number of radios that were in for repair.

The manager, a tall thin man, lived in a rather dreary apartment building in Union Street. He was married with one child, a boy of around six years of age and must have suffered during the Occupation. He had to support a wife and young child with no grown up adventurous boys and girls to help out by way of collecting firewood, gleaning, visiting the countryside, doing odd farm jobs and being partly paid in farm produce. How survival was possible, living in an apartment with no fires or stoves and reliant on an uncertain supply of gas and electricity is difficult to determine. Even in late 1940 and early 1941 our manager always appeared worried for by this time his job and livelihood were precarious. I imagine that he could only see hardship and deprivation ahead. At the time I was young, had no fear for the future and gave less concern for our manager than I am now voicing.

A teenager is a true philosopher for he makes use of what is going at the time and has little concern for what might happen within a day or two - certainly, no concern whatsoever for possible events six months hence. In those days, without the understanding or erudition for such things, I was a true philosopher and had much enjoyment from whatever was available. Despite the ignominy of being an enslaved people and in some fear of restraints on our freedom, the Occupation years were not the unhappiest of my life.

To return to our manager, when a load of batteries was too much for my bike, he often accompanied me on the deliveries riding a second delivery bike, a bike with a much smaller carrier. Being a manager, he had pretensions of gentility and wore his suit and tie. Trouser legs stuffed into his socks and ramrod, he looked incongruous perched on the seat of the delivery bike.

I left Foster's in May 1941 and did gardening and farm work until I joined Mr Dale's Boot and Shoe Store in Burrard Street in September as delivery boy and odd job lad. Mr Dale was a small, dapper, well dressed man with dark hair plastered back and a small black moustache. His wife, although a little plump, was also immaculate in her dress. However, the winner by far in style accoutrements and haughty disdain was their daughter Mavis.

The three of them served in the shop, although there was little enough to sell. Mavis was married. The husband, poor man, never appeared on the scene. She was in her mid-thirties, heavily made-up and a great gossip. Her place behind the counter was immediately in front of the fire which gave plenty of heat behind the counter but little in the shop overall - certainly none in the store behind the shop which was my domain. In dress and appearance I was the odd one out for I wore patched and darned clothing to work as such better clothing that I possessed was saved for the good times after work and in the holidays.

Mr Dale was fussy and petulant but I always did my work, rode the delivery bike in all weathers and, in that winter of 1941, often returned from some task or other with soaking wet shoes and trousers. In January and early February of the following year it was bitterly cold and Mr Dale, to his credit, gave me a pair of boots and a set of overalls. Mavis sniffed her approval when I first appeared. I was smart but with no pretensions to being better than I had a right to be.

The pleasure of the work were my visits to Summerland on Rouge Bouillon. It was a factory where the States employed young women to make clothing of various types, presumably with imports from France. The womens' ages ranged from eighteen to forty and there were more than four hundred of them. I was soon on waving acquaintance with all of them and close encounters of the flirty kind with about fifty. Not the Little Sisters of course! I was often there collecting items for Mr Dale's shop and helping him with his selection of leather hides for distribution to Jersey cobblers.

Selecting the hides was just the job that suited Mr Dale. He could look at them turned over (by me) ponder and deliberate. This would take half a day. He would clap his hands, seat himself with his cobblers list and bid me commence. I would lift a leather hide, turn it over when Mr Dale would rise, take a marking crayon and write on the leather - Le Cornu, St Ouen. This leather sheet was then put aside.

The next one, Smith, Val Plaisant; Houillebecq, St Mary and so on. I realised that his selection was heavy leather for the country parishes and light leather for the town. There could be as many as fifty hides and we often spent three days to finish the work. The hides had to be rolled and tied and this was the worst job of the lot.

After instruction by Mr Dale, I laid the hide flat on the ground. A length of rope with a noose at one end was placed under the hide, then the length of hide was rolled and knelt on, one end of the rope being threaded through the noose and knotted. Mr Dale left after three or four had been tied to his satisfaction.

It was a strenuous, knee bruising business. However, it was not long before the girls came to my aid. They would help in the bending and rolling and, one either side, would sit on the roll whilst I tied the knot. Of course, there was fun and a lot of play when the work was in progress. A hide would jump free and straighten out and the girls would fall off the rolled hide with much giggling and laughter. They shared their odd bits of food with me, teased me and, to a large extent, mothered me.

I listened to their sometimes bewildering chatter. 'Jack's a pig.' 'Fred's smoochy!' 'Did you see the dress Beryl was wearing today? There's a swastika on her knickers, I bet.' Great bursts of laughter followed.

During those lunch breaks a group of ten or twelve gathered in a room near the leather store and discussed all and everything. 'Did you see Ginger Rogers?' cried one, jumping to her feet and running her hands down her skirt to her ankles. 'A beautiful long dress, if I had a dress like that, I bet I could dance like her. She was tall, blond, pretty and not unlike Ginger Rogers. She then twirled round and round, her skirts flying and showing more than was good for a boy of fifteen to see!

One of my declared admirers, a lady called Lavinia of thirty or so, who never ceased teasing me, would often come up to me and, to the amusement of all her co-workers, would put her arm around my shoulders and say very loudly: 'Give me a kiss Dickie my love' and pursed her lips in imitation of a split watermelon. It was of acute embarrassment to me and worse was to follow. Sometimes when I passed groups of girls one would call out 'Hello Dickie my love!' All would then burst into fits of giggles.

The leather hides arrived from France every two months or so and Mr Dale was the chief unilateral distributor of the Jersey cobblers' leather ration. I asked why the hides had to be rolled and tied. The answer was that they were mainly collected by bike and could not be handled in their flat state.'

The winter of that year was extremely cold. I did not have gloves and suffered from chillblains to both hands on the finger joints. These tended to split, due - as Mavis informed me - to putting my hands in front of the shop fire, disturbing her and being seen, heard and in the way. The girls at Summerland muttered and called shame on Mr Dale. Maybe that was the reason he gave me boots and overalls.

Mavis and Mr and Mrs Dale were not to be compared with their youngest daughter, Doris. Doris worked in a greengrocer's shop in Midvale Road. Her overalls and hands were almost always dirty by reason of her job, handling muddy potatoes, swedes and the like. She was a pretty, unassuming young woman and I quite enjoyed my chats with her when I either delivered something or collected vegetables for her parents. During winter, she and her girl assistant always had a saucepan of vegetable soup simmering on the shop kitchen stove and they always gave me a mug of soup when I called. Perhaps because there was neither meat nor chicken in the soup, it was always flavoured with thyme. To this day I am always reminded of Doris and the greengrocer's shop in Midvale Road when I smell thyme. The shop is still there, at the top of Midvale Road, just before the Rouge Bouillon junction. Thyme has not changed it!

All in all, Mr and Mrs Dale, together with Mavis, were not unkind and my visits to Summerland and the treasure trove of the big store at the rear of the shop made life enjoyable. This store was mainly shelved and under bottom shelves and in cobwebbed nooks and crannies I found all sorts of things. Cobbler's tools, shoe and boot laces, pairs and odd ladies shoes, tins of polish and dubbin.

Mr Dale was delighted to the extent that one day, wearing overalls, he joined me in a thorough search of the store. We unearthed more of the same and some walking sticks, an umbrella and, in a far corner behind a stack of broken shelving, so covered in dust and debris as to appear part of the wall that they had been placed against, we found at least a dozen pairs of boots and the same number of overalls. Mr Dale gave me some boot laces and two tins of dubbin. The dubbin, he said, would completely waterproof my boots. He was right. We congratulated each other and were both highly satisfied with our mornings work.

By early spring the shop closed at 2pm and I was free for the afternoon, unless a supply of hides had been delivered to Summerland. Such supplies became more rare as the war progressed. Work became less and less as supplies dwindled and long periods of no supplies whatsoever developed.

Idleness is a devil's weapon and my first show of bravado as far as the Germans were concerned had its roots in little to do on winter afternoons. I had remarked to friends that it would be easy, when riding a bicycle, to kick a German officer on his backside and get away with it. All that was needed was to choose a quiet road on a slight incline, select your man just as he is approaching a corner, ride past with your left leg extended, kick him, then peddle like fury round the corner and then away. He, the victim, could not shoot you as you would be around the corner before he could un-holster his pistol. For such big talk I was made to pay the consequences. You would be too frightened to do any such thing, they said. So, of course, I did.

The subject would not go away and the deed had to be carried out. A fine late spring day was chosen and Don Road at the junction of Francis Street the chosen site. Solitary German officers were plentiful coming from, or going to wherever German officers were wont to go in St Helier. Less than an hour's wait was needed, when our officer appeared on the left side of the road, walking towards the town. He did not look too grand, although he did have a pistol secured to his belt. With heart racing and fearful trepidation I mounted my bike, rode down Don Road, gathered speed, left leg out and, bang, my boot made perfect contact with his bottom.

My foot came to an abrupt stop, the bicycle carried on and I fell in the gutter. The officer was frozen with shock for many seconds. Then he swung round and saw me sprawled in the gutter. He shouted and presumably swore in German, gave me two or three kicks - but more prods than kicks. I scrambled to my feet and gave an excellent pantomime of the front wheel wobbling and me loosing control and crashing into him. The shouting and questions lasted some minutes but he was satisfied that it was an accident. He was hardly likely to believe that I had deliberately kicked him. He went on his way. Neither the bike nor I were damaged and I rejoined my friends with great satisfaction. I never tried it again.

In March 1942 my work with Mr Dale ended and I left the shop. The cowboys remained but I was the last of the Mohicans. I was never without work and during the spring and summer of 1942 I worked on small holdings and farms.

Fuel and food were now obtained with some difficulty but as a family, we managed. I never returned from the country without a load of wood and often I managed to get vegetables. My brother, Denis, was of the greatest help as, for long periods of the Occupation, he worked as a milkman or a baker. My father worked in a market garden and, therefore, there were generally some vegetables available.

My eldest brother, Middleton, had joined the Navy in 1938 and it was a great worry and distress to my parents that they were unable to receive news of him. He was, in fact, killed in Hong Kong in 1941 but they were unaware of this until after the war in 1945. There were and still are two younger sisters: Jean and Marion.

My father, Middleton John, called Jack by almost everybody, was hard working, educated - which he tended to ridicule - domineering at times, quarrelsome and staged his life way below his potential.

My mother, Mona Agnes (née Le Gallais), was of old fashioned, lady-like habits of both dress and manner. My elder brother, Middleton (Middi or Middy) was possibly her favourite child and he was always on her mind throughout the Occupation. She was unaware of his death until after the Liberation in May, 1945. The news of his death put her into a state of shock which lasted many weeks and denied her any joy of liberation.

Mother was born in Guernsey in 1899. Her father, Francis Le Gallais, was a Jerseyman who had moved to Guernsey in the early 1890s. He had married an Irish lady who had been a school teacher. Mother was Irish in appearance to the extent that she had bright blue eyes and black hair. My exploits must have given her cares and pain and when I was arrested by the Germans in 1944, her situation was little more than pitiful.

Neither of my parents overly interfered with my exploits against the German occupation forces. They, the Germans, were the enemy and the fine line between patriotism and juvenile delinquency was impossible for them to define. To me, of course, it was patriotism but well flavoured with excitement and adventure.

During July and August I worked on a farm in Grouville. The farmer's name was Joe Perradun - or a name very similar. I was employed for the harvest. The crop, mainly wheat, was cut by hand with a sickle then bound into sheaves and stacked in groups, like wigwams. These were later collected by the wagons and taken to the thresher which would have been previously placed in a convenient location on the farm. The work was hard but I enjoyed it. Working on the farm we were relatively well fed, always potatoes but with pork or ham, meat stews and plenty of bread and butter. We often worked late and care had to be taken to get home before the curfew.

About six of us worked on the farm during this period of harvest, Joe, the farmer, an Irishman called Paddy(of course) Hibbits, a southern Irishman, myself and two or three others.

Joe, a taciturn, almost surly man was short but broad and strong with plenty of hair to the sides of his head but none on top. He would work beside us for hours, seldom saying a word. His wife, on the other hand, was a garrulous lady, plump, cheerful and good natured, slightly taller than Joe. Joe called his wife Ma and we all addressed her as 'Mrs Ma,' with which she seemed content, for she never suggested that we call her anything else. What her Christian name may have been, I have no idea for it was never disclosed. Her chatter was incessant and a smile, a nod, 'yes' or 'no' was enough for Mrs Ma in her conversations with any or all of us.

During these occasions, we all became silent taciturn men. For the few days each farm required the Thechet, the threshing machine, was moved from farm to farm. Always in a hurry as there were many farms but few threshers. Upon arrival at Joe's farm, we worked from dawn to dusk. The thresher came with crew members, two of whom were in the dangerous position on top of the machine, feeding it with corn sheaves. Loaded wagons were pulled alongside and three of us stood at the corn stacked wagon, pitching sheaves (by means of pitchforks) to the men feeding the machine. The three pitchers developed a rhythm, 123, 123, so that the three sheaves should not land at the feet of the feeders at one time.

A most amusing incident occurred one day when we were threshing. Mrs Ma was on the wagon with the pitchfork, pitching corn sheaves onto the thresher when a mouse ran up her trouser leg. She dropped the fork, clutched her thighs and started screaming and yelling for someone to help. Joe was not immediately about and on the wagon with her was a man in his mid twenties and myself. The mouse appeared to be moving about in her trousers and her situation was desperate.

She made up her mind in an instant, most likely thinking that a boy was more innocent than a twenty-five year old man. I was yelled at to put my hand down her trousers and get the mouse out. Her hands still occupied in protecting herself I had to loosen the waistband of her trousers as the legs of the trousers were too narrow for entry in that direction and insert my hand trying to locate an animal, small and furry, that may bite. I thought that I had found it immediately but a kick and a yell, 'Lower! Lower!' told me that I had not. I got it at the back of her leg, just above her knee, in clutching her trousers she had trapped it there. I gripped it, pulled it out and threw it across the field.

She composed herself immediately, fastened her trousers, called for Ben, the oiler, to find two pieces of string, which were handed to her and she tied the bottoms of her trousers. The incident was closed! Not so for the rest of the threshing party as snorts, gasps, giggles and occasional bursts of laughter continued throughout the remainder of the day.

After that day and for many days to follow, I was the butt of every joke anyone could think of, except Joe and Mrs Ma. She blushed occasionally when I looked at her but I was innocent at the time, had little or no carnal knowledge and the incident had been an embarrassment to me. I never discussed it with the other workers although I was teased and questioned. Mrs Ma realised this and I became her favourite.

Paddy Hibbits had become a good friend during my stay at the farm. He was a simple, naive man who worked hard and with no special interests outside the farm. He surprised me one day, in a discussion about the war, by saying that he supported Britain in the war. He noticed my surprise and told me that of his Irish acquaintances in Jersey, support for either side was roughly split down the middle - fifty percent for Britain and fifty percent for Germany. I am certain that he really did support Britain as, had he done otherwise, that would have been the end of our friendship. I was, like all my friends, patriotic, even if carelessly so.

As the work eased off in late August, at around 4.30pm we would go to Paddy's room. Its approach was through a straw littered barn, up wooden stairs, through lines and lines of boxes filled with seed potatoes, to a door at the west end of the barn. On opening the door, one walked into a very pleasant room. Two windows, one to the south and the other to the west, overlooking the farm yard, the rear of the farm building and the farm kitchen. The room was furnished with bed, table, bookcase, two armchairs and a table with two chairs. It was curtained and carpeted, if a little threadbare, both were clean and bright. The three granite walls were distempered in white and the studwork partition between Paddy's room and the barn was painted blue, with a simple 2'6 x 6' plywood door painted red. I congratulated Paddy on his upholding the red, white and blue'. It was a pleasant, comfortable room. There were no toilet facilities however, other than a bathroom-type washbasin mounted to the south wall with a shelf above where Paddy's washing things were kept. The toilet and showering facilities were downstairs near the exit of the barn. These were communal to the farm-workers. However, none of the other farm workers were resident at the farm and, working in the fields, the great outdoors was more convenient. Paddy, in the main, had the place to himself.

The wash basin in Paddy's room had neither tap or waste. A bucket filled with water was placed under the basin and, to wash, the basin plug was inserted in the plug hole and the water in the bucket poured into the basin. Washing completed, the bucket was placed under the basin, where the waste pipe would normally be. He would pull the plug and the bucket took the used water. Paddy told me that he occasionally made a mistake and pulled the plug, forgetting to place the bucket under the basin. He told me this story with great glee as, on one such occasion, he was dressed in his best trousers and shoes as he was going to church with Joe and Mrs Ma for an old farm worker's funeral. He pulled the plug and his shoes and trousers were saturated. He could not go in his second best which, insofar as he had best and worst, with no in-between, he went with wet shoes and trousers and caused more giggles than are seemly at a funeral.

We talked of Ireland, farms, horses and racehorses, the war and what we should do after the war. I had no real idea myself but in the meantime I told him that I had taken dance lessons and liked dancing. He was enthusiastic, jumped to his feet, selected a record from a small stack on the bookcase, wound his gramophone, an old fashioned instrument with a great, bell shaped horn and played his favourite song. He played it over and over and on future visits and was the only record I ever heard him play. Some sixty years later, I can still remember the tune and the opening lyrics. 'One two three Faden' cried he, 'You're quite a fairy but you have your faults. Whilst your left foot is lazy, your right foot is crazy, Faden McFaden, I'll teach you to waltz.' After the fifth playing, Mrs Ma called us to tea.

Paddy, a man of between thirty-five and forty, very fair skinned, his face in summer always a deep red, was a very kind man. You could

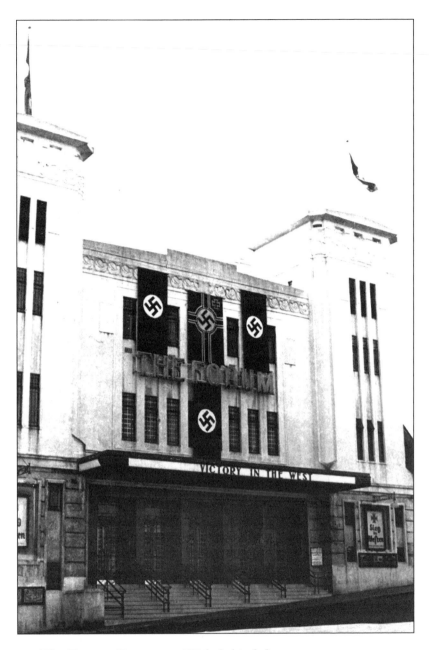

The Forum Cinema on Hitler's birthday
shows *Victory in the West*.

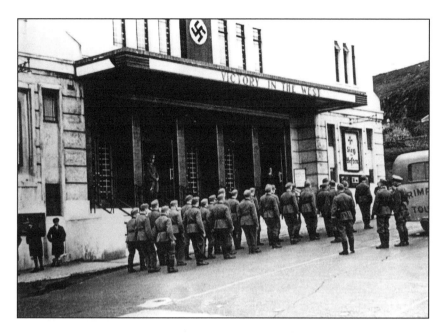

Above: Troops arrive, Note the sloping car park.
Below: German Military Orchestra performs.

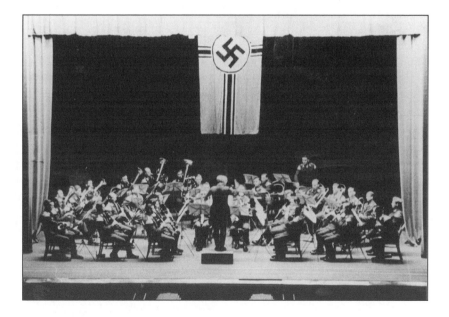

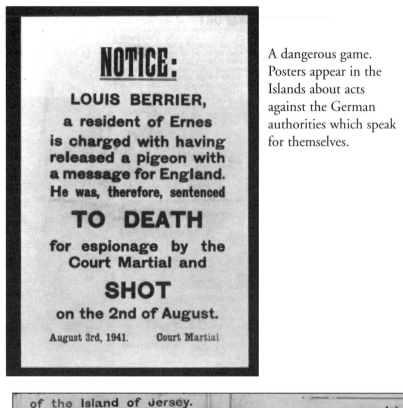

NOTICE:

LOUIS BERRIER,
a resident of Ernes
is charged with having
released a pigeon with
a message for England.
He was, therefore, sentenced

TO DEATH

for espionage by the
Court Martial and

SHOT

on the 2nd of August.

August 3rd, 1941.   Court Martial

A dangerous game.
Posters appear in the
Islands about acts
against the German
authorities which speak
for themselves.

of the Island of Jersey.

1st July

All Inhabitants must be indoors by 11 p.m. and must not leave
their homes before 5 a.m.
We will respect the population in Jersey
attempt to cause the least trouble, se
taken.
All orders given by the Military Auth
obeyed.
All spirits must be locked up immediately
supplied, obtained or consumed hence
does not apply to stocks in private house
No person shall enter the Aerodrome a
All Rifles, Airguns, Revolvers, Daggers
other Weapons whatsoever, except So
with all Ammunition, be delivered at
12 Noon to-morrow, July 3rd.
All British Sailors, Airmen and Soldie
Officers, in the Island must report
Office, Town, at 10 a.m. to-morrow
No Boat or vessel of any description,
Boat, shall leave The Harbours or any
same is moo without an Order from
to be obtain Commandant's
Boats arri must rem
leave,
The crew
the Harbo
Sale of Motor Spirit
Delivery of Food
Military Author
The use o
Black-out Re,
ks and Shops
order to confir
at 11 p.m.

To the Chief of the Military a

BEKANNTMACHUNG:

FRANÇOIS SCORNET,
geb 25-5-1919, zuletzt wohnhaft in
Ploujean (Departement Finistère) ist
wegen Begünstigung des Feindes durch
beabsichtigte Unterstützung Englands
im Kriege gegen das Deutsche Reich
durch das Kriegsgericht

ZUM TODE

verurteilt und am 17-III-1941
erschossen worden.

Das Kriegsgericht.
Den 23-III-1941.

PUBLICATION:

The population is herewith notified that
FRANÇOIS SCORNET,
born on May 25th 1919, residing in
Ploujean (Department Finistère) has
been sentenced

TO DEATH

by the German War Court and has
been shot on March 17th, 1941. This
had to be done, because of his favouring
the actions of the enemy by wilfully
supporting England in the war against
the German Empire.

German War Court.
March 23rd, 1941.

7 Every host ction
ollov d b bardmer
c se of eful surr,
peaceful habitants ar

sentativ

roperty,
antee'd

not admire or express a liking for anything he had without him seriously pressing you to take it. I never expressed a keen desire for his McFaden record - poor Paddy if I had.

He helped me in gleaning, in breaks, or when a daylight hour was free. This is a backbreaking tedious job. It consisted of picking, by finger tips, grains of wheat or oats that have fallen to the ground. A half pound of grain an hour would be a very good result. With the two of us, we sometimes managed two pounds at a series of gleaning sessions. He was delighted if we managed two pounds or more and distressed when it was a meagre half pound or so. I took the gleanings home and we turned them into flour by grinding the grains in a hand type coffee grinder.

I left the farm in September. I visited Paddy two or three times thereafter and we were always given tea by Mrs Ma. Our friendship faded as my visits ended. This, in part, was due to my bike tyres wearing out with no replacements available. I did try a garden hose but it was a difficult and bumpy ride and the garden hose tyres did not last above ten to twenty miles.

The Germans' visit did not end. They remained much in evidence and their restrictive orders and proclamations became more and more oppressive. To a large extent, the States of Jersey did not exist, for as a governing body, we knew little or nothing of their activities. The same would apply to the Jersey Police. Little was seen of them and even less known of their duties. The Germans ruled and controlled. An event in early 1942 would indicate the general tendency of our thoughts and from time to time, our resentment and desire for revenge.

My involvement in a major plan of sabotage occurred in very early 1942. The Germans had taken over the Forum cinema in Grenville Street. In the forecourt was an asphalted car park which was constructed on an incline from a high at the rear, bordering La Chasse, to its low point where it connected with Grenville Street. Often, ten to fifteen German officers' cars and two or three lorries for transporting troops were parked there.

At that time, I had become friendly with a lad named Peter Hassel - how or why I do not remember, most likely from the swimming club. We frequented a café in Grenville Street just before the corner joining Colomberie on the Forum side of the road. This café was a meeting place in the winter months for young people, most any time between four and six in the afternoon.

The plan was simple, slink among the cars - unscrew the petrol tank caps, place a length of hose pipe into the petrol tanks of four or five vehicles at the rear of the carpark, a suck or two at the hose ends and the petrol would then flow on to the asphalt, down the slope to the gutter in Grenville Street. The petrol would flow down the gutter to a drain just before Colomberie where we would wait with a box of matches. Flames would race up the gutter, across the car park to the open petrol tanks. Explosion after explosion and the whole group of vehicles would be destroyed. That was the plan.

We cut five lengths of hose pipe and one wet evening we put the plan into effect. Fortunately, we lost our nerve at the last moment. Resolution faltered and we reduced the number of cars to two, one each, placed the hoses, got the petrol flowing, then re-grouped at the Colomberie drain. Sure enough, it worked perfectly, very soon a multicoloured stream of petrol, flowing over the water in the gutter, reached the drain.

We watched for some time, then decided that it was too dangerous, local people would be hurt and the Forum and surrounding properties might well be set alight. We went back, removed the hoses, replaced the petrol caps and threw the hoses over the wall bordering La Chasse. The only outcome would be two German officers running out of petrol on their way back to their quarters.

The rain was light and with five hoses in five petrol tanks, the scheme would have worked but the danger to local people and reprisal by the Germans, which would have been harsh, made us change our minds.

We did not leave empty handed, for we managed to open some of the cars. I obtained a German Officer's brief case and a swastika. Inside the brief case was a folded document which, when opened out, showed the silhouettes of British and German warships as seen from an aeroplane. The car owner must have been a *Luftwaffe* officer. The swastika had eyelets at its four corners and would have been secured to the top of a car.

Some few months later Peter Hassel was to make an attempt to escape by boat to England but was caught. He and his friends were later deported to Germany and a prison camp. He was a brave, good lad.

CHAPTER 3
THE BEECHES FOR EVER

In September, 1942, I returned to school. I entered De La Salle, a Catholic boys school taught by the Brothers of the De La Salle Order. The school's common name and most often used was 'The Beeches.' How my parents managed the fees, I do not know, for they were by no means wealthy. Some sacrifice to their comfort must have been made. I have been told that the States gave assistance as shortage of work for young people required some alleviation by means of keeping them at school. The ordinary States schools, like St Luke's, had no facilities for children much over fourteen.

De La Salle was situated - and still is - near the top of Wellington Hill: 'Wellington Heights' of the school song. The school in those days consisted of the School House where the Brothers and occasional borders lived and a row of six classrooms in line along the East side of the upper playground. Their entrance doors led directly onto this playground which abutted the lower playground and was both longer and wider and at a lower level and formed the western boundary.

The Masters were: Brother Edward, Brother Marcel and another Brother whose name I cannot remember and in that order of priority. Two lay teachers, one Mr O'Shea and another with whom I had little connection and whose name now escapes me. There were also two recent ex De La Salle boys who worked with the juniors. I was in the fifth form. There was no sixth form. We were not clever enough or perhaps it was our ages. We were all sixteen and under and the total number of pupils in the region of 120.

Brother Edward and Mr O'Shea attended to my education and, all in all, they were likeable men but their eccentricities are a fillip to memory. Brother Edward's form of punishment was unusual. The week's ill-doers were called to the fifth form classroom. A week's   takings' would, on the average, be ten. We were lined up in front of his desk and read the history of our misdeeds, of our stupidity and of his grave doubts for our futures. During his recital, which lasted for ten minutes, he waved and gesticulated with a long, pliant cane. He struck no-one but newcomers were soon to be made painfully aware of its purpose, for on the conclusion of his lecture, often in mid-sentence, he would rise quite suddenly to his feet shouting 'Get out of my sight you good-for-nothings,' rush around his desk and chase us to the door, lashing out with the cane.

Of course, there was a great scramble for the door and the old sinners would escape scot-free as they were prepared and ran for their lives as soon as Brother Edward jumped to his feet. The slower and the newcomers received repeated whacks to their bottoms. This finale spoiled any seriousness of the occasion for we giggled and laughed as we scrambled to escape the cane, falling over each other to get through the door and often tumbling onto the upper playground in a heap of waving arms and legs.

Brother Edward, a plumpish, rotund man, was a good teacher and I probably learned more in my two years at De La Salle than I ever had before. He had his oddities but these were few as, apart from the chase with the cane, I can only remember his afternoon summer naps as being odd. After prayers, for prayers were quite the thing at De La Salle, Brother Edward on a warm afternoon would nod off and, if we were very quiet, he would sleep for half an hour.

It was on one such, very hot afternoon that a farmer's son named Hedley crept out of class and returned with three bottles of cider. Most of us took a few swigs and soon became giggly and jokes were exchanged. The resulting noise awoke Brother Edward, who, looking at our flushed faces and noticing our unsteady movements, immediately sent us outside to sit in the shade. He thought that the heat was too much for us. We did no further work that day and were sent home early.

Mr O'Shea taught English and Literature. He was a slim tallish man with slightly sunken features and deep set eyes and, of course, an Irishman. It was rumoured that he was not trained in any given profession and had obtained his position by some subterfuge or other. As had many men like himself, he must have suffered during the Occupation, for he was married with a very young child. My understanding of his worth was based upon a reasonable premise, as literature was my best and favourite subject and the only subject in which I could do well in exams. Mr O'Shea also had a penchant for literature and, in his own fashion, taught it with some flair.

Mr O'Shea in one of his exam papers posed the question 'Who was Shakespeare's favourite actress?' On reading this, I put my hand up and, when noticed, I told Mr O'Shea that he had made a mistake with this question as there were no female actresses in Shakespeare's time. He thought for a moment, gave me a token clip and said that I must be the stupidest boy in the school. Of course, it was a trick question and now everyone knew the answer.

The next day when he read out the results of his examination, he started by saying that he owed me an apology. I was not the stupidest boy in the school but only the second, as a boy named Somany was the stupidest. His answer to the question had been 'Miranda.' Two things intrigued me about this episode. (1) In the introduction to one of Shakespeare's plays, the writer had said that Miranda was Shakespeare's favourite female character. I thought that Somany was better informed than he appeared to be. (2) Had Mr O'Shea misunderstood his own question and Miranda was meant to be the answer?

I liked (Tim) O'Shea and once, during some nastiness over a collection of some sort, a boy named McGarry made some accusations against Mr O'Shea. These were later proved to be ill-founded. However, there was distress on the face of the accused. I defended Mr O'Shea by standing up and telling everyone in general and McGarry in particular that he was a sorry idiot and should be sent to two or three of Brother

Edward's sore bottom chases. McGarry said he was not. I repeated that he was and the argument ended with the days lessons and nothing further was heard of the matter.

The Brothers may well have suffered grievously due to the Occupation but help was always to hand. Farmers' sons brought packages which were delivered to the School House and, from time to time, a horse and cart would turn up and Brother Edward would excuse himself from the classroom for fifteen to twenty minutes.

We, some of the older boys, would also help. We pushed and pulled a great handcart belonging to the school and in the charge of the school handyman. He was a small, thin man, another Irishman named Declan and might, at one time, have been a jockey. He was in his fifties so that his career over the sticks would have been long before the war. His conversation was superior to his work output and was always of horses, grand stables, the Grand National and a filly called Annabel. Until this time and previously, without giving the matter much thought, I always assumed that Annabel was a horse!

Well wishers of the school would call on the Brothers with offers of firewood and if the location was reasonably close to the school, volunteers were requested and four or five of us, together with Samson, our private name for the handyman, would push the cart to a wood or field, load up and trundle back to school. In either direction, up Wellington Hill or down Wellington Hill, gave problems, for pushing up was very hard work and holding the cart from running down and away had its difficulties.

Sometimes we collected wood from demolished outhouses and once, passing through St Saviours Road with a particularly good load, a German officer stopped us and demanded to know where we had obtained the wood. This we could explain without fear of any wrongdoing.

Then he demanded that we take it to his quarters in a large house across the road. We refused with great indignation. This was Brother Edward's wood and we explained that Brother Edward was a priest and that the sanctity of the Church forbade us to hand over the wood. We spoke and almost believed that it was the Pope himself that we were defending. The officer, nonplussed and in some confusion, waved us on our way. We did not shout and dance until we were well out of sight.

There were, of course, causes for trials and tribulations outside of school and on one fine afternoon in early September of 1942, a school friend and I went to Mount Bingham where we were to witness acts of open rebellion against the Germans. The Germans were deporting a large group of local people, both of Jersey birth and of British birth. I was particularly concerned as a girl named Doreen was being deported with her family and at the time I was sweet on Doreen.

Mount Bingham was the nearest we could get to the docks but the whole of the dock area was clearly visible from Mount Bingham hill. More and more people arrived at this vantage point and by the time we could see the deportees being marched up the Albert Pier, some two thousand people would have been crowded together from the foot of the hill to the top at La Collette.

There was much anger as the group to be deported were the third or fourth such group and disgust and fury was in everyone's hearts. Caution had been disregarded and resentment had boiled over into outright defiance. Insults were shouted at German guards, every patriotic song known was sung. Slow hand claps, stamping of feet and every resource used to show contempt and disgust for these mindless ruffians who were the cause of needless pain to entirely innocent victims.

A covered lorry arrived which, as the road was impassable, came through Mount Bingham Gardens, backed as close to the road as it could get and when the rear cover was removed, a machine gun and machine gun crew could be seen, the gun pointing at the crowds. The temper of the crowd was such that even those in the machine gun's sights ignored it and continued yelling.

A group of German officers appeared and, through a loudspeaker, ordered the crowd to stop and go home. In the great tumult of noise very few heard and none complied. The officers made the mistake of sending troops into the crowd in an attempt to regain order. Fighting broke out. German troops disappeared into the fringes of the crowd where blows and kicks were exchanged and when they reappeared, in retreat, they were bloody with uniforms torn and wore the sheepish air of defeat. Perhaps their first!

They re-grouped near their officers. The whole of the Mount Bingham Hill was packed with people. Those at the foot of the hill, some one hundred and fifty yards from the crown, would be unaware of the lorry-mounted machine gun, but armed troops had appeared on the Mount Bingham escarpment, looking down at the crowds. Their elevated position meant that they were clearly visible to all and although there must have been some apprehension that the machine gun would be used no one seemed to care.

The officer in charge was most likely in a quandary. He was reluctant to kill one hundred civilians without orders from the top and therefore did nothing.

I managed only one punch at one of the German troops, as everyone in the vicinity had the same idea and I was brushed aside. A Frenchman named Barbier was shouting great oaths in French, fighting his way through to the Germans in the crowd and punching and kicking for all he was worth, which was quite a lot for he was a big, strong man and filled with bloodlust. He had to be restrained from following the troops when they retreated. Another man, a youth appropriately named Killer, broke a tennis racket over a German's head.

The end was theatrical, silence spread through the crowds, the deportees were leaving the ship and were walking towards the Weighbridge. It was unbelievable, it must be untrue and silence reigned for minutes until it could be seen to be real. The deportees were away from the ship and soon out of our sight. Great waves of cheering echoed again and again from the cliffs of the Mount. Good tempers and cheerfulness replaced the anger and frustration. The crowd quietly dispersed whilst the Germans stood their ground but did not interfere - the riot was over.

My friend and I left without let or hindrance and I thought that everyone had been allowed to leave unmolested. It was only later that I heard that some few were arrested among whom was Barbier but I understand that, considering the event and the complete disregard for German authority, they were dealt with lightly. That the Germans did little more than heavy handedly bluster, is perhaps not difficult to understand. The officer in command would need orders to open fire and such orders might well require instructions from Germany. It was better to do nothing!

I had to make my way from Mount Bingham to Rouge Bouillion where, in a nearby side street, Doreen lived. My way was largely barred and I had to go down to La Collette and up Green Street and through the town. By the time I reached Doreen's house she had gone out and, as I was informed, with a boyfriend. I am not very lucky at cards either!

When we returned to school the Mount Bingham rebellion was discussed for days. Most boys wished that they had been there. School life went on. We discussed the news for we were well informed, being experts at making crystal radio sets, or rather, we became experts by trial and error. All that was needed was: a coil, an ear phone, a whisker and a crystal. A piece of coal would often work as a crystal. The coil and the earphone were the most difficult to obtain. It was a tedious job winding an insulated length of wire into a coil but the earphone was impossible to make ourselves. They had to be found. However, needs must when Adolf drives.

We discovered that in many old houses, the servants call system contained coils. These were located in the indicator boxes mounted on walls in the servant quarters. The indicator boxes had a display panel indicating 'study' or 'drawing room' or even 'front door.' Old houses were plentiful and many unoccupied. The earphones were even easier to find. German field telephones were just the thing. The sets were a bit scratchy and faded in and out but they worked well enough.

Making crystal sets became an annual event, rather like marbles. Without rhyme or reason, once each year it would be marble time. Someone would turn up at school with marbles and the marble season was in full swing to last for two weeks, then disappear until next year. It was the same with crystal sets, roughly every mid October it was crystal set time.

Our time at school, considering the circumstances, was not entirely wasted. We studied, played sports and even pretended to learn German. This language, on the orders of some German authoritative imbecile or other, became compulsory. In our opinion, to learn the language would be unpatriotic, so we gave very little attention to it. The Brothers must have been of the same opinion for they did not press the matter. Little known to the Germans, they had a saboteur in their midst, for Mr O'Shea was to try his talents at teaching German and succeeded to the extent that we learned nothing.

From time to time a German from their propaganda department attended classes to check on our progress. If he got any satisfaction from his visits, it would only derive from conclusive evidence that the Germans were far more clever than the British. In absolute exasperation he informed us that in all his years of education he had never met with a stupider group of boys. He was never to change his opinion. Two or three of the more studious boys showed interest in learning the language but a few threats convinced them to be as stupid as the rest of us.

A large part of my popularity at school was most likely due to the fact that I played water-polo for the Beeches Old Boys team whilst still

a junior. My immodesty stems from the fact that I was voted in as House
Captain of Stanley, one of the four De La Salle houses. The previous
Captain had left school and an election was called.

The boys of the house voted and the result read out by Brother
Edward in the fifth form classroom. The votes were almost evenly split
between myself and another boy called Stephens. I won by seven or eight
votes. Jock Harris received one vote and Brother Edward, in reading this
out, looked across at Jock. 'You voted for yourself Harris.' Jock hotly
denied this and Jock was in fact innocent.

Brother Edward called me to his desk, handed me the House
books and records. He remarked that he thought the voters had made a
mistake in electing me. However, my popularity intrigued him and, not
entirely for my own comfort, he was to take more notice of me from that
election day on.

I had, of course, made a lot of friends at De La Salle but of special
note were Donald (Don) Bell and Francis (Jock) Harris. Among this trio
Don Bell was a lad of some substance, for he had de-railed a German
train. The Germans at the time were building rail lines in all directions
but mainly confined to the South and West of St Helier. These were
used for carrying building materials for the sea defence walls and gun
bunkers. Not too far from Don's home, near Red Houses, the Germans
had constructed a main line with a series of spurs. The main line had
been completed but the spurs had not and, except for twenty yards or so
of track, the rail line ended.

Having watched the train movements and examined the
switching equipment, a long steel handle with a cylinder of solid steel at
the top of the handle and the base connected to the switch gear of the
rails, Don noted that the handle, lifted up and swung completely over,
changed the set of rails from the main rail track to the spur track.
Waiting in the trees for the sound of an oncoming train, Don had darted
over, swung the switch gear handle to connect the main line with the
spur and ran back to hide in the trees to watch the outcome.

Along came the train, pulling a number of wagons and on reaching the spur junction ran along the spur until it ran out of rail. The engine was travelling at around fifteen miles per hour. It cleared the track taking five wagons with it and ended up on its side in scrub and sand. There was great shouting and cursing and, as far as Don could understand, the Germans were blaming one another for the mishap.

A rail mounted crane would be required to move the engine and wagons. Don removed himself from the scene but from day to day kept his eye on it. It was four days later before the main line was again in use. The switch gear handles were removed, now presumably carried on the engines and further and similar sabotage was not possible.

Our first major act of reprisal, later to be called a 'raid' was the armoury at the Merton Hotel on Belvedere Hill. Jock had noticed the armoury and had investigated the possibilities thoroughly. This armoury was perfectly placed for a raid, for it was at the corner of the Merton at the top of Mary Lane. Running from Georgetown, this lane joined Belvedere Road. The window to the armoury in Mary Lane, was a steel framed multi-glass paned structure.

Jock had noticed that one of the glass panes was loose and could be easily removed. Both the lane and adjoining road were little used and there appeared to be little or no insurmountable difficulties. The glass was frosted and Jock could not see the contents of the armoury but he assured us that it was full of good things.

We were careful and watched the armoury for some days as our main concern was German soldiers, mainly officers, coming and going. We noted that on their exit from the Merton main entrance they invariably turned left towards the town - in the opposite direction of Mary Lane and the armoury window fifty feet around the corner. Plans were made and the deed was soon to be carried out.

A little after dark on an early spring evening, we raided the armoury in Mary Lane. The lane was about three hundred yards long and could be ignored as far as danger from that quarter was concerned for anyone entering the Lane from Georgetown could be seen long before they reached us. Belvedere Hill was a problem as anyone entering the Lane from that direction would be immediately upon us. Therefore, one of us had to keep watch on Belvedere Hill, one had to stay in Mary Lane immediately under the entry window and one had to climb inside.

We tossed for it. Jock was to watch on Belvedere Hill, Don was to stay outside under the window and I was to enter the armoury. We carefully removed the loose glass pane and by pushing a hand and arm through this opening, found and swung the catch, the window opened. I climbed in and Don closed the window, the idea being that if someone appeared on Belvedere Hill, three taps on the window, Don and Jock would disappear and whoever was passing would see nothing amiss and would pass by.

It was a piece of cake as, on entering, I immediately saw a rack of rifles in the half light, grabbed three, knocked on the window, passed the rifles to Don, then climbed out. We closed and locked the window, replaced the glass pane, put the rifles in sacks we had brought with us and away. We had obtained a Todt forage cap which I had left in the armoury. We thought this a clever subterfuge as we were given to understand that there was little love lost between the *Wehrmacht* and the *Organisation Todt*.

Whether it worked or not we never knew but it most likely caused some confusion. We all reached home safely. Jock and I lived within a mile or so but Don had to ride his bike to St Brelade with the rifle in a sack tied to the crossbar.

I was much later given to consider the hardening of minds and lessening of fear that this type of raid, repeated again and again, instils in the raider. Familiarity breeds contempt! This first raid at the Merton Hotel was carried out with fear and trembling, whereas six months later we would have taken our time, looked over everything on display and chosen whatever it was we fancied. However, at the time we were happy with the rifles, treated them as favourite toys and soon understood their simple yet deadly mechanics.

At school, the following day we were exuberant, discussed it with some pride and much satisfaction. We told no other boys for we were aware of German informers and, although we had no doubts of the boys themselves, they might talk with outsiders. We followed the three monkeys' advice.

My school life continued through to 1944. My two years at De La Salle were not entirely wasted. Mr O'Shea gave me a great liking for literature and gratuitously, he came to share my opinion. We played cricket and football on the lower playground and had sports days, held on the same lower playground.

Both cricket and football had their restrictions with respect to lost balls on the south side of the playground. A Carmelite Nuns' garden bordered on the south side and it was forbidden to penetrate a very dense, high hedge into their garden. As an austere Order, they did not chatter as most women would and it was impossible to know if they were in the garden or not.

Rules are rules but lost balls, almost impossible to replace, must be found. Certain adventurous boys volunteered to fetch a lost ball and this entailed painstaking, gentle progress through the thick hedge and parting the foliage in search of Nuns. The area immediately behind this hedge was mainly open and, if no Nuns were about, the ball might be easily found. If there were any Nuns around, a silent retreat was necessary and the game was over until the next break.

On the one and only occasion when we were noticed, we were noticed in dramatic fashion. A large heavy boy, Ozouf, a farmers son, tripped over branches at the fringe of the hedge and fell into the Nuns' garden. We heard the crash and then cries and screams. The vow of silence was broken!

Ozouf crashed back through the hedge and we beat a hasty retreat, hoping that nothing more would happen. Of course something did. A priest of the Carmelite Order called upon Brother Edward and we were all in a sea of troubles. No one would admit to this outrage and no one would tell on the culprit. We were all culprits in one way or the other and some six or seven of us had been major culprits at some time.

The troubles lasted for weeks and the lower playground was out of bounds for all ball games. Not being a Catholic, the seriousness of the matter escaped me until the many lectures and the stern, almost fearful looks of the Brothers made me realise that something quite bad had happened and I, in turn, was frightened, although of what I did not know.

As all good and bad things do, the matter faded and went. The only good result was that the caretaker had found some chicken wire. The support posts of the fence, high steel angle iron separating the nuns' garden from the school, were still in position and only replacement chicken-wire was required. Ladders were found and half the fifth form happily assisted the caretaker but everyone was as quiet as a dumb mouse.

It is a well known fact in Jersey that if by happy chance you pass a man of regal mien and manly grace, he is almost certain to be a Beeches Man. Thank you, De La Salle at the top of Wellington Hill. May you prosper always.

CHAPTER 4
THE POOL

The pool of this story is the Jersey Swimming Club premises at Havre des Pas on the outskirts of St Helier. The club was founded in 1865 and the present bathing pool constructed around 1900. It was and is three quarter moon shaped with an overall swimming area in excess of three thousand square yards. Most of this area is in deep water. At high tide the pool is covered and at low tide the pool retains its full capacity of water. There was a tower of diving boards, from thirty feet at the top board reducing in height to a fifteen feet board and a ten feet board combined with a springboard.

The pool buildings included changing cabins, cafeteria, terraces and stores. These buildings were approached by way of a steel columned timber decked bridge leading from the Havre des Pas road. In the summer time during the Occupation any number of between sixty or seventy members would be found in the late afternoons at the pool. The subscription was seven shillings and sixpence per annum, or the equivalent in Occupation marks.

During the summer months I spent every free daylight hour at the pool. In times of shortages and some deprivation it is interesting to note that the pool remained open throughout the Occupation. I note from club records that I scored two goals in a water-polo match for the Jersey Swimming Club team against the Beeches in 1941 and was in the Beeches Old Boys team which won the Occupation Cup in 1943 and in the same team in August 1944 when we lost.

There were many notable members during the Occupation whose fame lives on in the Pool Year Book. Of the young members some few would one day be lawyers of repute, the effect of excessive amounts of sea water perhaps?

Of the older members of particular memory are Mr Ching and Mr Croad who were close friends. Mr Ching was a plump, jovial man whose aim in life was to cheer everyone up or scold them into good humour. Mr Croad, despite his friend's best efforts, was a thin rather sombre man as suited his profession. Mr Ching was a tobacconist and Mr Croad an undertaker. Their friendship caused no untoward comment at the time but today it might be said that Mr Croad had all the advantage of it!

In summer the pool was the centre of all our activities. On Saturdays and Sundays we seldom went anywhere else. We, of course, were constantly swimming, played water-polo, talked and played. Do not ask how, with such short rations, we were able to swim for hours and play water-polo which is a most strenuous game but we did.

The pool was not just a swimming club but also a social club. The girls had some strange notion that boys and girls should be paired off. They selected who should be this or that girl's boyfriend and, with very little option on the part of the boys, a choice had been made and that was that. This could be a three monthly event and a boy could be chucked by the girl. It was commonplace for the boy to take very little more notice of his selected girlfriend than he had before his selection. I was often chucked for great dereliction of duty, for none were Indian Princesses.

Playing water-polo for the Beeches Old Boys team while still a junior, I had a certain popularity in the pairing activity of the girls and often was chosen by one of the prettier ones. The main purpose in the scheme of things was for the girl to be your supporter in the water-polo matches. There were three or four teams, all local. The Germans never played and, if they had wished to, we would have had to abandon the matches.

Of these teams, the Jersey Swimming Club team and the Beeches Old Boys team were the strongest and the greatest rivals. The girls would watch the games and cheer for the team in which their boyfriend played. These water-polo games gave rise to much enthusiasm and, in certain months of the summer, were the centre of activity at the pool.

The pool was not used very often by German troops. From time to time an officer would walk in and, less often, other ranks. They would walk about, perhaps sit for an hour, then leave. There was the utmost indifference to their presence and if any thought was given to them, it was merely a wish that they would go away. At the time I never gave any rational thought to their feelings about being treated as lepers by a very large majority of the local population and it must be assumed that some isolation was felt. Even today, without any conscious resentment, I tend to avoid Germans and, when their company is unavoidable, eye them with the suspicion a policeman eyes a suspect.

Happily, they never went swimming, unless forced to do so and, occasionally, a group of fifteen to twenty would arrive for swimming lessons. Their normal instructors were an officer and a sergeant for whom swimming and swimming lessons were very basic. Their methods were amusing to watch and their practice of what they called *execution* was astonishing. A pole with a length of rope tied at one end and a harness at the end of the rope was strapped to the learner, who was then made to climb the ladder to the ten foot board, stand at its edge over the water and, at the sound of the officer's whistle, jump.

In the water the victim struggled and floundered until the sergeant, by lifting the pole in the air and with parade ground shouts of instruction, ordered him to swim. Even in the Third Reich, orders were sometimes disobeyed. Half supported and half in desperate fear, with kicks and splashes, the ladder at the pool side was reached and the half drowned victim climbed to safety. Their swimming lessons were of no use whatsoever and were more than likely to give the men a great fear of the water. It certainly did not teach them to swim.

On one such occasion I was sitting at the edge of the pool with

Percy Gosling and two other lads watching the swimming lessons about fifteen yards or so away from this scene of activity. We had ceased to remark on the lunatic methods of German swimming instructions as we had seen it often before. However, we watched and an event occurred putting us all in a serious predicament. In jumping from the ten foot diving board, the harness, attached to a German soldier, had come loose and, without support, he hit the water, disappeared for some seconds and emerged with flailing arms and choked calls for help. He was drowning!

None of the German swimming party made any effort to dive in and save him. This was, of course, understandable with respect to the learners but neither the officer nor the sergeant made any useful effort other than to shout orders not to drown. They were both fully dressed including their jackboots but their coats and boots could have been quickly removed. Perhaps they could not swim?

We watched the soldier drowning. What to do? He was an enemy and it was not our patriotic duty to assist the enemy. He, the soldier, was near to being a dead man when, with one accord, we dived in and with no difficulty brought him ashore. He was unconscious. The German soldiers crowded around but it was immediately obvious that they had not the slightest idea what to do. We took charge. We rolled him on to his stomach, arms half bent above his head, which we turned to one side and checked to ensure that he had not swallowed his tongue, then Percy pumped him dry. This we had been taught in life saving training and the method used was to place both hands on the victim's back, thumbs almost meeting at the spine, fingers curled down to the ribcage. From a kneeling position one leaned forward with all ones weight transferred to the hands, then leaned back and repeated this exercise until water flowed from the mouth. In this case, a fair amount of water gushed from our patient's mouth and within a minute he was gasping and retching.

We indicated a towel and made rubbing gestures but as the officer spoke a little English we were able to tell him that the man needed a good rub down, to be covered and kept warm. We then left them. An ambulance with a doctor and medical orderlies arrived twenty minutes later.

Soldiers were sent to search for us and we were brought to the medical officer who spoke good English. He thanked us and wanted our names and addresses as he said that some official recognition of our help in saving a German soldier's life would be made by the concerned authorities. We, of course, refused, as we wanted the whole incident kept quiet. After some argument, he shrugged his shoulders and they all left. Other than from pool members, we heard nothing more of the incident.

Although unlikely to be because of fear of swimming lessons, one German soldier committed suicide at the pool. This happened in mid summer of 1943 and came to our notice by a sudden frantic excitement among the Germans attending swimming lessons. The Germans used the upper row of changing cabins which, in better times, had been the ladies changing cabins. The German soldiers were all dressed ready to leave when it was noticed that one was missing. They searched the changing cabins, one door being bolted on the inside, they broke in and found the missing soldier. He apparently had stabbed himself with a bayonet and was dead when discovered.

We watched in silence as an ambulance was called, the body carried down the concrete steps and placed on a stretcher, then carried through the pool, along the bridge to the ambulance waiting on the Havre des Pas road. We were all silent and rather upset. The poor fellow must have been in great distress - maybe he was to be sent to the Russian Front.

As a group at the pool, we were perhaps carefree but not unaware of outside events. Most of us had access to a radio, if only a crystal set and were able to discuss the situation and our day of liberation as none of us had any doubts of eventual victory. We discussed the Germans and the fortifications that they were building all over the place and the slave workers employed in this work. We were concerned and gave such assistance as we could which, in the main, consisted in tossing apples and cooked potatoes into their working areas. We thought them all to be Russian. This was not so, but gave rise to a schoolboy joke: 'Are you Russian?' 'No! I take my time.'

The German Army appeared to be a mixture of the old and the new. Tanks, guns, troop carriers were much in evidence but also there were many horse-drawn wagons used by the German troops. These wagons had a single shaft and two horses harnessed at either side. The shape of the wagons was odd, very German in our opinion as they had a sort of triangle shape, much wider at the top than at the bottom so that the appearance from the front or rear was V shaped and the sides sloped in from the top to the base, therefore the floor area of the wagon was a great deal less than the top of the side panels. These trundled all over the place - generally heaped with sacks - most likely food supply wagons. I did not like the Germans much but I did like their horses.

'Jerrybags' were, from time to time, a topic of conversation when some girl or other whom we knew was seen walking out with Germans. I knew of no harm caused by these girls and their behaviour may be excused on the grounds that they were, in the main, girls in their mid-twenties at which time of life in normal times they would have flirted and been courted. Local men of their own age were few and one must suppose that nature would take its course. They were not numerous and suffered a certain amount of abuse and, to my knowledge, suffered in silence and did not complain to their German boyfriends.

One such was a girl I knew well and one day, passing her on my bicycle, I saw she was walking with a German officer. I called out 'jerrybag!' and rode away. Two days later I was called to the Police Station where her father worked as a sergeant in the Jersey Police. He took me to an interview room where I received the worst reprimand I had so far suffered. He told me that his daughter's and his family's business was none of mine, I had very much upset his daughter and I was lucky that she was a good girl and did not make a complaint to the Germans. In all good faith, I agreed with him and offered my apologies to both himself and his daughter. He was mollified and sent me away, advising me not to do it again. I did not, as I was sorry. To cause pain at such times for the idlest reasons was not the action of a Pukka Sahib.

It was from the pool, early one summer's evening that we carried out one of our more foolhardy exploits. We rowed out to a German motor barge shipwrecked on a group of rocks some two miles offshore. We used two floats with paddles. These floats were two cigar shaped wooden hulls with three deck planks screwed to the hulls at front, rear and centre. They were approximately twelve feet in length and five feet wide overall and very low in the water. We had two of them and had got them from one of the German occupied hotels. My mind says Tam's Pantry at St. Brelade but I cannot remember or conceive how we were able to carry them from St Brelade to St Helier without being noticed as the use of such floats was forbidden by the German authorities.

These floats had been stored and restored in the unused basement of my house in Don Road. As we were taking the floats from Don Road to the Pool, by pure mischance, while removing them from the basement, up the basement steps to the street, just as we came out from the front entrance gates on to the pavement, a German naval officer almost fell over the float, due to our sudden appearance on the pavement. He, of course, stopped us and told us that the use of such sea-going craft was forbidden and if we had taken it to the shore we would have been in serious trouble.

We thanked him profusely for his help and advice and took the float back in. Fortunately, the second float had not appeared and he had not seen it. Giving the naval officer fifteen minutes to get well out of the way, we carried the floats to the pool - about a mile away - and arrived without further trouble.

Placing them in the water, they sank. They were never to be truly buoyant until we had opened up the hulls and placed sealed paraffin cans inside. They were hidden in a little used storage area of the pool, were never remarked on and might not have been further used had the Germans not, so opportunely, shipwrecked a motor barge on the Demi des Pas reefs.

We had noticed the shipwreck some days before and four of us - myself, Jock, Jacques and another whose name I forget - launched the two floats just as the tide, on the flow, was approaching the pool wall. Two to each float, we paddled off toward the Demi des Pas rocks where the German barge was high and dry but as the tide was coming in it would not be high and dry for very long. The journey was a difficult one as we had to follow channels among the rocks which curved and turned and our approach to the wreck was by way of a series of zig zags.

On our approach, the tide had risen considerably and was flowing around and over the many rock outcrops causing eddies and small whirlpools. We had no fear for, with the possible exception of Jock, we were all excellent swimmers. It was daylight but as we were very low in the water and among rocks, we were not clearly visible from the shore if any real watch was kept. However, German discipline has its rewards for unless the German soldier was a fairly high ranking officer or had been specifically instructed to watch the seashore, he had neither the inclination nor the authority to take any action.

We eventually arrived at the shore-side of the reef where the barge was marooned. Two were left to look after the floats while Jock and I climbed the rock face, four or five feet in height, to peer over and note our best approach. We were nonplussed, a German E boat was anchored in deep water not more than two hundred yards from the wreck. The purpose, no doubt, to stop pirates like ourselves hoisting the skull and crossbones on our prize.

We climbed back aboard the floats and discussed what we should do and decided that we should wait, hoping that the E boat would up-

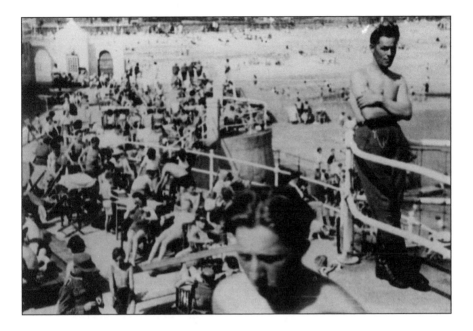

Above: Havre des Pas Swimming Pool in 1943.

Below: The Pool remains in use today.

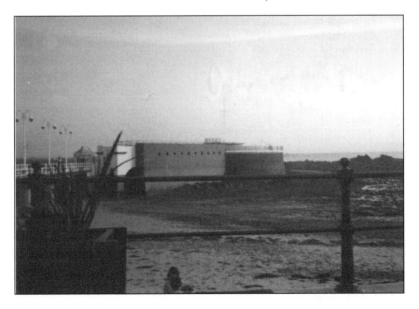

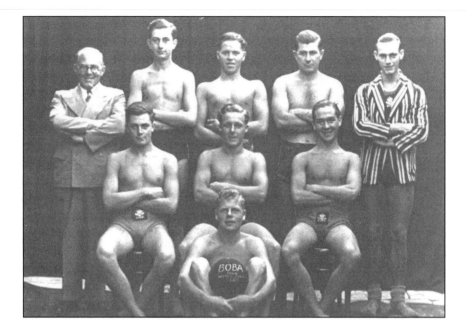

Beeches Old Boys Water Polo Team - 1943
(from top left)

Bert Liron - Soleil Levant
Raymond Vitel - fight with guards
George Abbot
Bob Cornish - Bob's garden
Don Nicole - Colomberie House
Bunny Vitel
Percy Gosling - Helped to save the drowning German soldier
Roy Cuquetel - Deportée, Glmort
Me - with ball

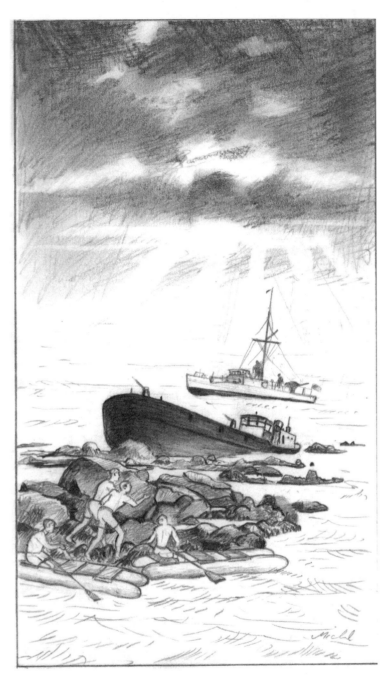

On to the shipwreck- Pirates all

anchor and leave. We could not wait indefinitely as the rising tide would raise our floats above the reef and we should be in full view of the E boat's crew. Ten minutes later, we were within three feet of the top of the reef and would have to leave within three or four minutes.

Peering over the reef, we watched waves breaking over the wreck and, to our joy, heard the engines of the E boat come to life. The Captain must have considered that no one could board the barge with the tide on the flood and was leaving the scene. The E boat gathered speed and was soon around the Dogs Nest and out of sight. We had minutes to spare, so two of us scrambled across the rocks to the wreck which was rising and falling with much screeching as its steel plated hull was scraping against the rocks.

We managed to board and looked into the open hatch of the hold. It contained and was almost filled with what appeared to be fine granular coal dust but of greyish-black colour. There were bicycle parts strewn over this dust and two or three dozen bottles of Cointreau. We jumped into the hold not more than three feet below the hatch, grabbed four bottles of Cointreau each, placed them in the sacks we carried, - our burglars loot bag - and then back to the floats which were by now a matter of inches below the reef.

To anyone not familiar with the great tidal surges of the Channel Isles, with a variation of tide levels of thirty to forty feet, the return journey would have appeared impossible. By habit we had become careless and the danger only added to the excitement. Paddling through channels in rushing water, the tide coming in so fast that every minute saw waves breaking over rocks above us like a waterfall, soaking us and threatening to wash us off the floats, we headed for he shore.

However, our return journey was much quicker than the outward one, as the tide had covered a large part of the rock reefs and we could sail in a more direct line. We paddled over the pool wall, now entirely covered by the rising tide, hid the floats away and celebrated with a swig of Cointreau each. None of us were drinkers and one swig was all we wanted. The remaining bottles, plus one with an inch missing, we shared, two each. My parents were not drinkers either and the Cointreau lasted for ages. Some did find its way into the carrageen moss jelly at Christmas.

During the winter months the pool crowd broke up and except for one's closer friends, we saw little of each other. The exception being the pool dances of which there were three or four each winter and the Forum was the venue until this was completely taken over by the Germans. To prepare myself I joined Miss Le Feuvre's Dance Academy in David Place. For sixpence a lesson, the waltz, slow foxtrot, quickstep and tango were available.

Miss le Feuvre was a tall, thin lady of indeterminate age. She was addressed as Madame and addressed the pupils, of which there were between six to ten at each lesson, by their Christian names. A session lasted forty five minutes of intense application. Presumably by Madame's prior arrangements the boys and girls were almost always evenly divided.

We applied ourselves happily enough but insofar as the majority were new to dancing, the first three or four lessons were a series of toe crunching, entangled legs and red faces. The girls picked it up more quickly but very soon, chided and encouraged by Madame, the part of the brain that controls leg acrobatics clicked in and followed, one after the other with tolerable grace.

I attended the last group of the day, from 8pm to 8.45pm. Madame was interested and kind and she often continued until 9pm. As we improved, Madame's enthusiasm increased and with encouragement and insults she turned us into Ginger Rogers and Fred Astaire. 'Brian, you are a young man, not a duck! Dickie, she is not a bear, she won't eat you, pull Doreen closer! Come, I'll show you.' With my nose an inch away from Madame's bosom as she was a good nine inches taller than me, we danced the waltz. An unlikely Fred Astaire, whereas Madame, in her movements, very like Ginger Rogers. Madame was graceful, her body pliant and, once over the initial embarrassment, dancing with her was easy and pleasurable. Some four shillings and sixpence later, I was a credit to Madame, to the waltz and quickstep, not so good at the slow foxtrot. The tango remained incomprehensible. However, I was ready for the dance.

My first dance was New Year's Eve 1941, held at the Forum. The dance was held in a ballroom on the upper floor between the twin towers. Over one hundred dancers attended and the dance started at 7pm and ended at 10. We all had a glorious time and for a few short hours we twirled and pirouetted and, remembering Madame's admonition, I pulled all the girls closer.

Our pool season started early and ended late. Some of us would always turn up in April and were still there in October. Mr Cooper, the maintenance and 'all things' man would let us use the pool, although it was not officially open in the early and late months. Swimming in October was fine for the water retained a reasonable temperature whereas April was merely a quick plunge and out, hardening oneself for May. However, at the pool it was always summer, the sun always shone and life had nothing better to offer.

CHAPTER 5
NEMESIS IN RAGGED TROUSERS

Following our raid on the Merton Armoury, it was necessary to find ammunition for our rifles. Don, Jock and I went on the prowl for a likely German store or armoury as it was a little too soon to return to the Merton. We chose, on the surface, the most unlikely target, the German Bunker on the South Pier which had been constructed on the base of what is now the St Helier Yacht Club. Its location guarded the pier heads from any allied attack from that direction. Our reasoning for considering this bunker to be a likely target was twofold: it was easy to watch for reconnaissance purposes and there were no German billets overlooking this bunker. There was some sort of naval quarters at La Folie Inn but this building did not overlook the bunker and, being naval, they had no great interest in army affairs.

The smaller German gun emplacements or bunkers were almost always constructed in the same manner. Although there were steel doors with gun outlets on the seaward side which were kept bolted until an emergency arose, there was always an entrance on the landward side. This comprised a steel or wooden door with a simple padlock.

In the case of this South Pier bunker, the landward door could be watched from Mount Bingham. We could, in complete safety, by looking over the granite wall at the bottom of Mount Bingham Hill, watch the bunker and time the movements of the German guards on their patrol. These guards, always in twos and armed with rifles, visited and checked the bunker and other German stores and positions on a timed routine. On timing them over some days, we noted that they would visit the South Pier every forty five minutes. They were as regular and precise as a train timetable and we learned the exact timing of their arrival at the South Pier. We came to know when to expect them and, sure enough, heralded by the sound of their jackboots on the granite pavement, they appeared, on time. Often their jackboots could be heard long before they appeared and we were to consider the Germans lacking in imagination and almost entirely predictable when later during the Occupation, patrol guards covered their jackboots with felt so that their approach was unheard. However, since their timing remained exactly the same, their flash of inspiration was in vain. They were always in pairs, armed with rifles and adhered to a strict timetable which included a three minute stop at each structure under their surveillance. A rudimentary examination by flashlight, a smoke, a chat and away.

The raid was planned and executed on a darkish winter night. The patrol arrived at their appointed time of 8.15pm, left and would not be seen again until 9.00pm. The three of us scrambled down the steps, one hundred and twenty of them, from Mount Bingham to the pier, along the pier to the bunker back door.

We carried a jemmy, for we were professionals in our intermittent trade. The jemmy had been made for us by a blacksmith and was perfectly suited for the purpose required to be done. It was eighteen inches long, one end split into a claw shape and bent to within two inches of the shaft, the other end flattened to a screwdriver shape and slightly bent. Little could withstand the jemmy's physical power.

We reached the door, which was of steel, complete with hasp, staple and padlock. The jemmy made short work of the padlock and we were inside the bunker. We found treasure: rifle bullets, machine gun bullets, spare machine gun barrels, tins of chocolate, sardines, tuna, pork, sausage and sauerkraut.

We were away within fifteen minutes with sacks filled. We closed the door and replaced the padlock as, although broken, the steel swivel would fit into the body of the padlock and on visual examination appeared to be intact. We re-traced our steps, carrying the heavy sacks. Our business now was not to be noticed by German street patrols. It was not yet curfew but carrying sacks we might well be stopped, questioned and searched. However, we had devised ways and means as we always chose dark nights and whenever possible, rainy weather. The guards were not enthusiastic or bright and alert on such nights. When we heard them approaching, we dropped whatever we were carrying over low garden walls or even at the base of high walls. We would saunter past the patrol with no greeting sch as 'Sieg Heil' or 'Heil Hitler' which would be suspicious in the extreme and could only be derogatory!

When they were well away we would return and retrieve the sacks. It was almost always sacks - brown dirty bundles matching most night backgrounds. We made our way up Mount Bingham, down to La Collette and along Havre des Pas, where Jock lived, continued on to and up St Clement's Road to Don Road, where I now lived.

In this house in Don Road, there was a unused basement, where, in one of its rear rooms, was my store. Don and I, by means of the basement steps, entered the basement and stowed the sacks. Don lived at St Brelade and his share of the booty would be moved there small amounts at a time. He rode home with pockets filled with rifle bullets and tins of chocolate in the carrier bag of his bike.

The basement at Don Road was a great asset insofar as it was unused by none of my family but me. It was dirty and littered with old broken furniture and suffered from damp. The house was large, with basement and three upper floors. I had oiled the lock of the basement entrance door (located under the main door) and could come and go as I pleased. My store of trophies was to become a small armoury in itself as, at its peak, it contained:

3 rifles
1 revolver with only 6 rounds of ammunition
2 German soldiers uniforms, although I had no idea of which
regiment I belonged to, or for that matter, which two regiments.
2 machine gun barrels
1 crate of pineapple hand grenades
6 stick grenades

1 sword
rifle, machine gun and pistol ammunition,
miscellaneous cans of meat, fish, sausage and chocolate.

To put the foodstuff into the family kitchen was a difficulty I overcame by introducing it in small quantities from time to time. Questions were asked and vague answers given until the small but continuous supply went without undue comment. It was a way of Occupation life and some questions were better left unasked and unanswered. If familiarity did not breed contempt in this case, it became a normal course of events.

With rifle ammunition to hand, I could now play at loading and unloading the rifle. In a steel box, the width of a bullet and about one foot deep and eighteen inches in length, the rifle bullets were on clips. By pulling back the bolt, placing the clip in a groove at the top of a magazine (disclosed by pulling back the bolt) pressing on the top bullet of five, the five bullets entered the magazine and the rifle was loaded. Pushing the bolt forward and down, a bullet was fed into the chamber, the bolt locked in position and the rifle ready for firing. Lifting the bolt and pulling it back, the spent cartridge was ejected, push the bolt forward and another bullet was ready in the firing chamber. In my case, of course, live bullets were ejected.

Playing this game for days, the temptation became too much. The rifle had to be fired. One afternoon when everyone was out of the house, I went to the basement - this by way of a stairway entered by a cupboard-like door to the rear of the hall. The door to my basement room was to the left, immediately at the foot of the stairs. I entered, retrieved the rifle from under an old carpet covered with pieces of broken furniture, loaded and was ready.

With the door closed and a rag of a curtain across the half window, I aimed at the wall on the door side of the room and pulled the trigger. The noise was terrifying - a great bang - which the whole of

Jersey must have heard ringing in my ears. Slightly dazed, I quickly hid the rifle away, ran from the room, turned to dash up the stairs, then disaster! A large part of the stair wall had been blown out. The bullet had passed completely through the wall. Stone, plaster and masonry debris covered the stairs. I went upstairs for a shovel and brush and spent long minutes cleaning, putting the debris in one of the front rooms, the whole time in expectation of hammering at the front door. The damage was a two foot diameter hole in the wall for half its depth. It was at shin height when walking up or down the stairs and not entirely evident in the poor light of the stair area. It certainly did not look like a bullet hole. Where the bullet had entered the wall, there was nothing more than a small round hole which was easily disguised. The bullet had crossed the basement passage and entered the wall dividing the house from the next house in the row of similar houses. I prayed that it had not entirely penetrated, leaving a similar hole in the wall of the neighbouring basement.

I then did what I had intended to do immediately after firing the rifle - which was to run up the stairs, open the front door to enquire of excited neighbours where the shot had come from. There were no excited neighbours and the street was quiet, with the odd persons passing about their business. Very surprising but I suppose that the occasional explosion was not uncommon during the Occupation years and most people minded their own business where Germans might be concerned. Seemingly, next door did not have a two foot hole in their basement wall, for nothing was heard from them.

It will perhaps be noticed that we had no knowledge of ordnance in the early days of the Occupation and knowledge was only to be gained by trial and error. Jock was to badly injure his eye in attempting to dismantle a machine gun firing bolt and I had an idiotic episode with a hand grenade.

I was examining a pineapple grenade by turning it around in my hands. It ticked! In panic, I put it on the basement floor, threw an old mattress on top of it and sat on the mattress attempting to muffle the noise of the explosion. I sat there for a good five minutes, but nothing happened, so I again examined it. In turning it around, I noticed that the pull ring attached to the detonation pin fell against the casing as the grenade, which when turned, made a ticking sound.

We raided the South Pier bunker four times in all and another bunker at the sea end of Green Street three times. These raids would be months apart but it has since surprised me that the Germans made no special efforts for the protection of these bunkers. We watched for any untoward activity after a raid but noticed little different.

I have thought that whoever was responsible for guarding these bunkers covered up, for the damage was small and whatever we had taken was easily replaced. It would have been difficult for them to pin-point the time of the break-in. All guards would have been under suspicion and the officer in charge would be culpable. A cover up would be their only solution. These gun positions were unmanned but were ready in case of allied landings.

The Green Street bunker was not such an easy target as the South Pier. It was built into the Sea Wall with its rear entrance a few feet from the Havre des Pas and Green Street road junction. It was surrounded by houses and a building housing German officers was within one hundred and fifty yards. The entrance, forgetting the steel bolted gun housing doors, was through a tunnel leading to the concrete and steel encased gun platform. A simple timber door with hasp, staple and padlock, laid flat on the ground on top of a flight of concrete steps going down to the tunnel, was the means of entry. We, on this particular raid, had watched for some days, timed the guards and were confident that there was no real problem. Our confidence must have been exceptional as this was our third raid on this bunker.

On a dark night, raining, with the streets empty but for we prowlers of the night and distant German patrols, Don and I

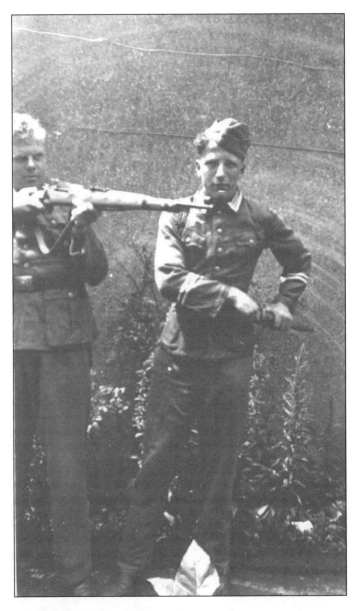

Me (left) and Jock in 1943 wearing our stolen German uniforms.

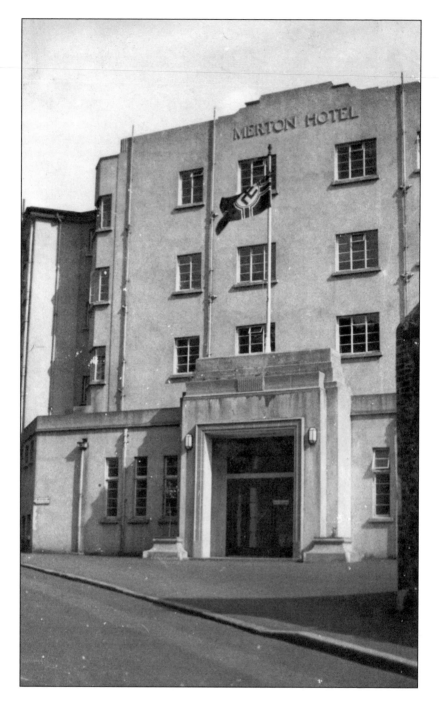

The Merton Hotel during the Occupation.

Mr. West's Picture Palace.

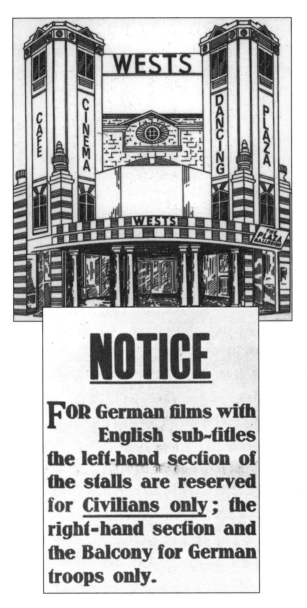

commenced our raid. We carefully ignored the padlock as, being a timber door, using the jemmy on the padlock tended to split and break the wood securing the hasp and staple. We therefore carefully pried the flat screwed section away from the timber frame so that it might be replaced as if still intact. We had gained in experience and were more and more careful. In this case our care was well rewarded. Further, our tactics had changed. Only one of us was to enter the bunker, the other to replace the padlock, hinge, hasp and staple as if undisturbed.

The gods smiled kindly on us that night. Insofar as it was my turn, I entered with two sacks and Don put everything in order on the outside. I went down the steps along the passageway to the heart of the gun position, loaded the sacks and away. We did not have torches, as batteries had long since been unobtainable, so I made my way by use of matches, feel and familiarity with this bunker.

In leaving the gun chamber, I had knocked over a field telephone and hoped that it did not connect with the officers quarters a little up the hill. I hurried to the trap door and as I reached the top of the steps, I heard boots on the gravel approaching the door. This was immediately followed by rays of light through the edges of the door and concrete stair-head. I was petrified and sat on the stair and waited for the worst to happen.

The torch light disappeared and a conversation in German started up while my head was two feet from the guards boots. Time passed so slowly but eventually I heard the crunch of gravel and the guards went on their way. I did not move until I heard a gentle tap on the trapdoor. I whispered in answer, the trapdoor was opened and we were safe. We replaced the door to appear undisturbed, as the guards needed some thanks. The broken door might not be discovered for some days. The field telephone almost certainly did not connect to the German officers quarters. Maybe it was disconnected. For once, the guards had been unpredictable for they had arrived a good fifteen minutes before their allotted time. Maybe it could have been a guard change. We never raided Green Street again.

Such a close encounter was to happen to me again at a later date but actual capture occurred, arising from my own stupidity. Raids or jobs were confined to the winter months. They were always planned, guards timed and familiarisation of place and area were a must. However, the following episode was neither planned nor given any rational thought.

On a clear March evening in 1943 I was walking along the Esplanade with a lad named Vitel. Our walk was aimless and in all likelihood we would have turned off at Castle Street, through the town and home. The time was about 8.00pm. There were many warehouses along the Esplanade at that time and our interest was drawn to German notices on double wooden gates leading to a yard and a warehouse beyond.

The gates and wall were five to six feet in height and were easily climbed, so, without hesitation, we climbed over the wall and into the yard. The perimeter walls of the yard were lined with rabbit hutches, complete with rabbits. These were of no great interest and attention was given to the warehouse. The doors were locked and secure. However, there was a window and entry would not have been difficult by that means. We had no tools with us and while we were weighing up the situation a German patrol arrived.

Vitel and I made a dive for the straw under the rabbit hutches in an attempt at concealment. This proved useless as there was little straw and the guards torchlight soon picked us up. There were two guards in the patrol, both with rifles. A few kicks brought us to our feet and, after some shouted questions and threats, understood by the facial expressions and not the words, which were unanswered and unanswerable, the guards led us away.

After locking the gates, one guard handed his rifle to the other and took us by the scruff of the necks and marched us down the Esplanade towards the Pomme d'Or Hotel. Whether or not that was the guards destination I have no idea. However, we thought so and some immediate, desperate action was necessary.

The guard holding us by our collars was extremely vulnerable, his hands raised to grip our collars, his body clear for a great punch into his solar plexus. Fortunately, I was to his right and my right fist was free. With all the strength I could command, I swung my fist deep into the guard's stomach. He was finished immediately. He fell to the ground, writhing in agony. The second guard was desperately trying to free himself from his and his fellow guard's rifle but he was far too late. The adrenaline was flowing and the cry of battle had sounded. We threw him heavily to the ground, gave him three or four hard kicks and we fled.

We ran for our lives. A short way down the Esplanade, we turned at Castle Street, through Charing Cross, up the back doubles, cut through Waterloo Street, down Beresford Street to West's Cinema. The town was in an uproar as far as the Germans were concerned. Whistles were being blown, shouting coming from all directions. The unheard of had happened. Two armed guards had been attacked and the attackers were loose in St Helier. Gott in Himmel! or Hallelujah! whichever side you were on.

Our predicament was soon to be desperate if we did not find some place to conceal ourselves until the hunt was abandoned or there were more people in the streets, the town being empty as there was little or nothing to do at night. We had run any which way in some panic and our escape route home would, by now, be cut off. We were in Beresford Street. West's Cinema became an obvious choice.

West's Cinema stood in what is now known as West Centre. It was a fine, tiled building with its main entrance in Bath Street through a curving arcade. There were emergency exits in Peter Street and that is where we headed. We often went to this cinema for free, as we, like squirrels, had learned to manipulate the emergency panic door to gain entry. In some panic we opened this door from the non-panic side, secured it behind us, crept up the stairs and sat ourselves at the rear as far from the picture-goers as was possible. We were in a state of some shock and whatever film was being shown, I had no idea then and have none now.

However, comic relief was to hand. The nearest people to us started to fidget in their seats and look about accusingly at their neighbours. A most dreadful smell was filling the air and from where it came, fortunately, was not obvious as we were some seats away from the occupied seats.

We were wearing rubber boots, wellingtons, stolen from a German store and although our trousers were outside the boots, there was little space between the boots uppers and the trouser legs. In the excitement and unable to stop for the needs of nature, or any other needs, Vitel had defecated, the result finding the easiest route, had fallen into his boots, mashed up in the running and was now wasting its sweetness on the cinema air. I started to giggle and Vitel joined in. Whether or not the smell became part of the overall cinema environment and by familiarity became unnoticeable, certainly agitation faded and ceased and we were left in peace until the end of the show.

We left the cinema with the home-going crowd. There were German troops all over the place but we managed to reach our respective homes without incident. I was, a short time later, to put this down to the descriptions given of us by the guards we had attacked.

Repercussions followed and I was later informed by a lad named Bisson that his elder brother, a young man with curly hair similar to mine, had been brought in by the Germans to an identification parade. He, the elder Bisson, was taller, heavier built and some years older than me. The guards description of us must have been exaggerated for Vitel was thin and I was not all that robust. Bisson came to no harm.

As a footnote, some weeks later I came face to face with the guard I had punched. I was on a bike in the town: he was on the same side of the road walking toward me and ten or twelve feet away. Recognition came to us both. He stopped and stared, I gathered speed and was away as fast as I could. There were other Germans in the street and a bit of shouting could have resulted in my capture but he did nothing and I can only surmise that he was appalled that such a young, not overly strong looking boy could have got the better of him and his fellow guard. His look - at first, recognition, then astonishment - told the story. I do not think that he reported it, possibly from shame. I heard no more of it from any quarter.

A very large German food store in Commercial Street was an easy target. It was located in an old timber warehouse and entry was gained by way of the roofs of adjacent warehouses - which were empty - and through one of the vents along the perimeter of its side walls. This store was so well stocked that I doubt if it was noticed that intruders had helped themselves. The difficulty of climbing out, over roofs and down to the ground level prevented any heavy load. One tin of butter was a prize, as these tins were in excess of a foot in diameter and six inches deep.

Nine months after our first raid on the Merton Hotel Armoury, we returned. The window had been repaired but putty is easily removed as was the pane of glass it secured. Opening the window, we were faced with rows of rubber (wellington) boots. We removed them, pair by pair, to gain entry but the shelves in front of the window were very deep and thirty pairs of boots were removed before we had cleared enough space to be able to clamber between the shelves. We placed the boots against the wall down Mary Lane in line like soldiers on parade.

On entry, we discovered that the building was no longer an armoury but some sort of first aid store. There were plenty of boots, stretchers, ward trolleys, first aid kits, gas masks, capes, medical kits and supplies. We took two pairs of rubber boots each, together with first aid kits. We re-secured the window by means of part replacing the putty but left the boots in Mary Lane hoping that local people would notice them and they would soon disappear.

A favourite place for us was a German clothing store in St Luke's. I had entered this store five or six times with different youths at different times. It was a play-house rather than a place to be raided. Entry was gained by way of the front garden and then around to the back. We got in through a window by removing a pane of glass, pushing our hand through and releasing the catch. After the first visit, we carried sticky paper with us so that we could secure the glass once inside. The store was heaped with uniforms, jackboots, socks, gloves and various items of soft equipment such as canvas packs, side-bags, pouches and the like. Articles of clothing were heaped to half room's height and if any Germans had visited this store we might have been well hidden under these heaps of uniforms.

Very occasionally a pair of grey trousers could be found among the almost one hundred percent green. Gloves and socks were all green. Gifts of gloves and socks appeared in the back gardens of local residents, thrown by us on our way home and some items of clothing were to be given to Russian slave workers.

Jock and I were to be in a little trouble at this same store at a later date and John Rault was to be seen there on one momentous occasions. Five of us were searching for grey trousers in one of the front rooms on the upper floor when a German lorry arrived. Four soldiers jumped from the canvas covered rear of the lorry and a sergeant and driver from the cab. The sergeant mounted the steps to the main entrance, unlocked the door, called to the soldiers who immediately commenced unloading and carrying bundles up the steps and into the store.

Their work was confined to the first floor so we were reasonably safe on the third floor It was early afternoon as grey was indistinguishable from green in the half light. The sound of jackboots on stone and floorboards ceased. The work was finished and a soldier's break of chatter and cigarettes as evidenced by the noise and the smell coming up the stairwell. Steps were heard on the stairs, most likely the sergeant on a tour of inspection. The room we were in was filled with clothing halfway to the ceiling, so we all dived for cover under the heaped trousers. The sergeant appeared to be merely glancing into each room for, on each floor the footsteps, sounds on the bare boards of the landing, were heard to stop for a few seconds, then on to the next doorway. Footsteps stopped at our doorway, and other than the noise being made by the soldiers below, it was deadly quiet. He sensed something and remained for several seconds. Fortunately, the noise below became a racket. His concentration broken, he hurried across the landing and clattered down the stairs.

Shouts were heard, then more clatter as they all crossed the lower landing, the door slammed and locked, they climbed back on to the waiting lorry and they were gone. Vastly relieved, we emerged from our hiding place and curiosity aroused, we descended the stairs to see what the soldiers had delivered to the store. A heap of S.S. backpacks had been placed against the rear wall of the front room immediately to the left of the main entrance. On hands and knees, so as not to be seen through the main windows overlooking the road, we examined the packs. They were black canvas with a very dark fur flap (maybe black bear fur?) We, of course, took one each.

John's claim to fame were his involvement in our War of Attrition, although he was disabled. His left leg was shorter than the right and he wore a boot with a three inch sole. John's only compatibility with German patrol guards was that he was heard long before he came into view. At night, he often carried a club - an Indian exercise club. This had been drilled and nuts and bolts inserted into the drilled holes. It was a fearsome weapon, though I do not think that he ever used it in anger.

He was not often with us as his disability prevented rapid retreat. Perhaps by way of compensation he, on a fine summer afternoon, dressed himself in German uniform, entered a 'German only' café in Colomberie, and ordered, drank and paid for a cup of coffee. Place and time had been notified as he wished his great triumph to be witnessed. He limped from Val Plaisant to Colomberie in full German uniform with complete disregard for badges and his emblems being almost certainly wrong, and notwithstanding his limp, and entered the café. He had chosen early afternoon when the café would be quiet. However, the wish was beyond measure.

When he emerged from the café, we surrounded him, and told him, (ordered him!) to follow us to Don Nicolle's house at the top of Colomberie near the Roseville Street junction. He obeyed, was loaned clothing, congratulated, fussed over, then limped back to Val Plaisant where he lived. His luck had been tried and had held. We did not think that it could last a uniformed return trip to Val Plaisant which was why we had insisted that he change at Don's house.

CHAPTER 6
LIFE GOES ON

The advent of autumn found me crying for the loss of summer and happy days at the pool, partings of the ways for many good friends. However, a circular route and we would meet again next summer. We sometimes met at dances and arranged entertainments, often passed in the streets and met winter friends in those same streets, for in those days every third person walking by was a friend or acquaintance. Cheered by the thoughts of a poet - *"If winter comes, can spring be far behind?"* I found entertainment where I could. Our friends, the Germans, or jerries or squareheads, Fritz, Adolf, Heinrich and all that lot were never far behind. They did provide entertainment but one could not always be on the prowl, jemmy in hand.

West's Picture Palace was a great source of entertainment for me. I sometimes paid and sometimes went for free. To overcome my shame, I paid when I could afford it and as, when going for free, I could not enter through the emergency exit in Peter Street until the picture show had started, I caused no loss to the owners in lost seat sales. All in all, I doubt the owners would have considered it a bad bargain.

The variety and quality of the films shown was perhaps limited and few were in English, but from time to time innocuous films like Laurel and Hardy were shown. In the main, the films were in German with English subtitles. From memory my top choices were:

Cora Terry: Cora Terry of the film's title was played by a beautiful German actress. From memory, she was dark haired and not blonde and therefore an unlikely Nazi heroine, but what she did or did not do I do not remember. I remember her beauty and due to my nine lovelorn visits to see her I almost learned German. I can remember one dramatic denouément:

'Sie sind Greta Terry?'
'Ich bin nicht Greta Terry, ich bin Cora Terry!'
Of course, I knew it all the time!

The Man Who Was Sherlock Holmes: This was a good detective film. Two private detectives who could get little or no business, had the bright idea to dress up as Sherlock Holmes and Doctor Watson, the pipe and violin included. Business boomed and one of their particular cases was the film story. From time to time they came across a middle aged, smartly dressed man in the German idea of the English style. Each time he came across these heroes he would burst into laughter. The denouément, which was perhaps obvious, was that he was Conan Doyle. Strange that the Germans would make film heroes of three very English characters.

Baron Von Munchhausen: This was an excellent film. I saw it over and over.

Notwithstanding all the foregoing, pride of place must be given to 'Bomber Squadron Lutzow.' The reason for its pride of place rests with the great excitement and chance it gave us to express our feelings when it was being shown. It concerned a German bomber squadron and their war starting over Poland, France and England. It was typical of its genre and had it not been German, it would have been quite moving. However, the fun came on its first showing when the squadron was bombing England. When one of their planes was shot down by a British fighter the whole of the local audience clapped and cheered. The Germans in the audience waited until a British plane was shot down and they clapped and cheered. Insofar as the film was to show the loss and sadness of lost crews, plenty of German planes were shot down and there was plenty to clap and cheer about. However, seeing that it was a German film and the Germans could not be defeated, the German audience had plenty of their own opportunities for retaliation. Each night pandemonium reigned throughout the second part of the film. News spread and on its third or fourth showing, West's Picture Palace was overflowing and the cheers, shouts and handclaps were deafening, I had to pay each time. Loyalties could be demonstrated and independence clearly established. How soon these events came to the notice of the German authorities is unclear but insofar as the film was taken out of circulation after the seventh showing, they - the Germans and the power they could muster - used their only option within those seven days. It is sad that the States of Jersey saw fit to allow demolition of Mr West's Picture Palace. It should have had equal status with the 'Alamo,' a monument to 'Jersey the Brave.'

Other delights were available during the winter months - with amateur dramatics as a major source of entertainment. The Opera House with its plays and operas was open throughout the Occupation. Music Halls in chapels and halls were of the greatest amusement. Palaces of Variety, although on a very modest scale, opened and closed and closed and opened throughout the winter months. A night's entertainment lasted ninety minutes with a fifteen minute intermission added on. There would be eight to ten acts of dancing, singing, comics and sketches. Stars were born, glittered and shone for a few months and faded with the advent of spring. There were a few prima donnas but I do not think that anyone was paid. The takings at three or four pence a seat were meagre but what there was went to charity.

I fell for a girl named Yvonne, a star. She had a very sweet voice and a song that was a favourite of most audiences was a song of Paul Robson - which seems at first strange - but she sang Lindy Loo with great sweetness and effect. This song concerns a mocking bird and opens - 'Lindy did you hear that mocking bird sing last night? Honey he was singing so sweet in the moonlight' and ends 'My Lindy Loo, I'd lay right down and die, if I could sing as sweet as that to you, my little Lindy Loo.' When I first heard the song (Yvonne on stage and I some fifty feet away as I was acting as doorman at this particular show) I fell, lock stock and barrel and was prepared to lay right down and die.

I never did get to know Yvonne: 'hellos' and 'good-byes' were our sole source for love. I wooed her from the stalls, gazing cow-like at the stage. Yvonne achieved some degree of fame for she sometimes sang at the Opera House. Her mother collected her after each performance, which was explained to me, kindly, when I first asked Yvonne if I could walk with her to her home.

Love laughs at locksmiths, so I devised a cunning plan. I would become an actor, a star! Knowing most of the producers of these shows and perhaps owing to the fact that variety acts were not as pebbles on the sea shore, I secured a part in a show where Yvonne was to be a main attraction. I rehearsed and practiced and was ready for the dress rehearsal when Yvonne would appear. Being an old trouper, she did not attend general rehearsals. She did not come as, unknown to me, her mother, weeks before, had informed the producer that Yvonne would not be available for his production. The show must go on!

My act was to portray the plight of a broken hearted milkman - which suited my feelings at the time. On the first night, shaking at the knees, I appeared on stage wearing a milkman's apron and cap, pushing a small milk cart complete with two churns and started to sing- 'I'm a broken hearted milkman from Paddington Green.' Sobs and sniffles accompanied the singing. My song related to my love of a girl on my milk round. Scraps are remembered. 'At the sound of my milk cans her face she would show. When I asked her to marry me she upped and she cried. To marry a milkman she didn't feel inclined.'" On this line of the song my prop was used, this was a large red handkerchief, previously dipped in water and throughout the song used to dab my eyes. A milk churn lid was removed and the handkerchief squeezed so that water fell into the milk. This was an in-joke and caused much laughter and applause at the time as milkmen were often accused of adding water to the milk.

I was a great success, whether because I was good or very bad I do not know - more than likely the latter for I was not asked to perform again. My stardom lasted for six nights. Yvonne left my stage and I was only to see her intermittently thereafter. I think that unrequited love suited me. I had tried the requited variety with no lasting success.

Dances were common during the winter and, on average, I attended them once a month, if not pool dances, the public dances, which were frequent. The venue would be a church hall. I was acquainted with most of the girls to be found at these dances but there were newcomers. I generally went with a friend and not a girlfriend as I had no particular attachment throughout the latter part of the Occupation.

I sometimes went with Jock and he had the most ingenious method of checking the beauty of a distant, possible dance partner. Neither of us had 20/20 vision and his long distance viewing machine was invaluable. This consisted of a card the size of a visiting card with a pinhole. Taken from the jacket top pocket, peering through the pinhole, beauty clearly defined.

I was told a joke of a lad, without Jock's machine, who crossed to a lady sitting across the dance hall and suddenly in front of her realised that the lady was rather older than he had expected. In some confusion, he blurted out the first excuse that came to mind - 'Oh, I am sorry, I thought you were my mother.' She crossly replied 'Can you not see that I am wearing a wedding ring?' I laughed ten years later.

We did some good works in giving away goods and clothing taken from the Germans. Chocolate was surplus to any needs I could fairly claim as reasonable and I had dozens of tins. The chocolate was of the dark variety but, melted in hot water with milk added, it was a very tasty drink. This chocolate was found in every German bunker. The tins were an inch deep and three inches in diameter. There were children in three or four of the houses near my house and they all became the recipients of tins of chocolate.

I could not just walk up and openly hand out chocolate. The gift had to be from an anonymous friend. My first 'Father Christmas' act came in late November. I went to a house in Don Road Crescent where I had often seen children come and go. Late at night, just before curfew,

I approached the front door of the house with six tins of chocolate, gently lifted the letter box flap and posted the first tin which fell with a great clatter to the floor. Footfalls could be heard approaching the door and, not wishing to be seen, I placed the remaining five tins at the base of the door and ran way out of sight. I had left a printed note with the chocolate - 'Silence is Golden.'

I disposed of thirty tins of chocolate in this fashion. I think that I improved on the content of the printed message but never better than 'Top Secret' and never worse than 'Mum's the Word.'

Once only we delivered clothing to Goose Green at Beaumont where the Germans had a Russian Prisoners Camp. These were slave workers who, poor fellows, slaved daily on German defence systems and, in particular, the reinforced concrete walls along vulnerable sections of the Jersey coastline. A rumour was widespread among us locals that when a Russian died at his work, the body was thrown into the wall under construction and concreted in. I seriously doubt this as the Germans had engineers on duty and the presence of bodies in the concrete would seriously weaken the structure. However, the odd such incident may well have occurred.

The clothing to be distributed was not difficult to find and the clothing store at St Luke's was raided for coats, trousers, gloves and socks. The coats were mutilated to the extent that buttons and shoulder straps were torn off. Bundles were made up to which chocolate and a few tins of meat were added. At dusk, approaching the Goose Green prison camp by way of Sandybrook, the bundles were thrown over the barbed wire fence as near to the prisoners' huts as possible. Whether the Russian prisoners could disguise the green was not certain but prisoners have their own ways and means and it was hoped that some good use was made of our bundles.

My work and duties at home were not neglected. The constant search for firewood was a never ending chore and timber was often found in unlikely places. On one occasion, during a blackberry hunt with friends from the pool, we were combing the hedgerows in fields above Ghost Hill between St.Aubin and Ouaisné when we came across a group of guns covered with camouflage netting. There appeared to be nobody about and, after watching for some minutes, two of us found that the guns were decoys. Under the netting were timber structures in a rough imitation of field artillery with the deception being enhanced by a telegraph pole as the gun barrel.

The telegraph poles were much too heavy to move but these decoys were made from many sections of different lengths and sizes of timber. Firewood immediately sprung to mind! We continued blackberrying but the guns were not to be forgotten. Over weeks the guns were dismantled of pieces capable of being carried home, leaving heavy sections and telegraph poles lying on the ground. Five pieces of German artillery had been destroyed!

Low water fishing was another means of subsistence. We searched the rock areas of the seashore at low tide for crabs, fish left in pools by the ebb tide, ormers and, very occasionally, limpets and carrageen moss. Low water fishing was a hit and miss business, both in the catch (as often little was to be found) and on the state of mind of the German shore patrols. These patrols were erratic with their favours as at times they made no objection and, at others, they prevented access to the shore.

Again, the patrol's period of duty might end when we were way out amid the rocks so that the relief patrol would shout, wave and, if not immediately obeyed, would send soldiers to herd us to shore like lost sheep. One could be smiled at going in and cursed at coming out. The catch that was always available was limpets and, to a lesser extent, carrageen moss, though perhaps catch is a wrong word, for neither ran away!

Limpets were almost impossible to digest so we only used them to flavour fish soup. A screwdriver type tool is necessary to pry them from the rocks as their shell, a circular pyramid shape, once touched, the creature inside sticks for dear life to the rock and cannot be removed by hand. It can live both in and out of water for, in the tidal movements of the Channel Isles, it is hours submerged and hours high and dry. Taken home, removed from their shell, well washed and hammered flat is the preparation to frying them in butter. In times of butter shortage - which was often - a pint of milk put into a quart bottle and shaken a very long time would produce enough butter for the limpets. They were fried, then simmered for an hour, the limpets removed and thrown away and the resulting stock used in soup. Revolting! Carrageen moss was a type of seaweed which, when boiled and drained off, produced a jelly which is supposed to have medicinal qualities. It is seaweedy of taste on its own but with fresh fruit boiled with it (or chocolate or sugar beet syrup) it is not too bad.

Sugar beet syrup during the latter period of the Occupation was to take the place of sugar. On one occasion, having purchased a hundredweight of sugar beet, the family spent the whole day making syrup. We had an old-fashioned copper at the house. This was a very large copper bowl set into brickwork with a fire grate underneath. Years before, this was used to boil a family's weekly wash. Making the syrup was expensive with respect to firewood as the sugar beet required hours of boiling.

The Germans helped out with this, for unbeknown to them, a shed in the garden of a hotel in Colomberie occupied by them had been painstakingly taken apart from the inside, so that it still stood when we had finished but would collapse in the first high wind.

The sugar beet was well washed and cut into pieces, thrown into the copper, gallons and gallons of water added, the fire lit and syrup making was underway. A continuous watch had to be kept as the water boiled away and had to be replaced so that the fire needed constant attention. Some hours later the copper was half filled with a black liquid. This was strained and put into bottles. Dozens of pints were then put into our store.

My father, like most men with gardens, grew tobacco. We would help him to string it up to dry where it stayed until it became a brownish yellow. He would take it down leaf by leaf, paint each leaf with sugar beet syrup, then roll the tobacco leaf into tight bundles, secured by a length of cloth. Some weeks later he was happily smoking his pipe. Cider and calvados were also available to the men but this was only available at rare intervals as only the farmers had the means of production.

My mother, poor dear, suffered most from the complete absence of tea which she dearly loved. I could get coffee fairly easily from various German stores or bunkers but never found tea. I was often to remain over-long (where I should not have been) in search of tea. I never did find any.

Sweets, fizzy drinks, biscuits, ice-cream were unobtainable. They had disappeared at the beginning of the Occupation. We never seemed to miss such things. There was, however, liquorice during the early part of the Occupation. A man, very aptly named a Mr Trueblood, kept a chemist shop in St Helier on the corner of French Lane and Bath Street. His shop and its contents were relics of the late 1800s. Both the shop and the window were filled with great jars, bottles and bowls of glass and ceramic, unguents, herbs and medicines, pills and powders in these ornate containers.

In one very large glass jar were many thick sticks of liquorice. These were most likely meant to be a laxative, not a child's sweet but young boys do not mind. In those early days threepence would buy one of these solid sticks and, with a little husbandry, would last a week. The shop, immediately opposite the Soleil Levant on the corner of French Lane and Bath Street, is still there, but the contents and Mr Trueblood are long since gone. Mr Trueblood is memorable as, with no customers inside the shop, he always stood at the shop door. A tall man, oldish and with a great mass of pure white hair, a sort of Fuzzy Wuzzy of the Northern kind.

Almost immediately across the street but slightly higher up toward Queen Street, Mrs Riggs had a small café. Her only claim to fame was her potato cakes which at one penny a time, satisfied the mid-morning hunger. The combination of potato cakes and liquorice were exactly right: one needed the other. Thinking of my daily intake of potatoes, I must have eaten in excess of two tons during the Occupation years, for which Mrs Riggs was not entirely blameless.

The Soleil Levant public house, opposite Mr Trueblood's shop, was owned by a Mr Bert Liron who was short, plump and bald. It must be assumed that Mr Liron also stood in front of his pub and exchanged views with Mr Trueblood. If so, passers by must have been reminded of Laurel and Hardy. I did not know either the pub or the owner, Mr Bert Liron, at the time of Mr Trueblood but was to know him very well much later during the Occupation as he was a coach for the Beeches Old Boys water polo team. At the time, the pub was closed as there was nothing to sell but in springtime we often met there to discuss tactics for the coming season.

At the top of Bath Street, at the junction with Queen Street and Snow Hill, was a chemist shop called Croix De Lorraine and during the latter part of the Occupation the Germans once displayed in the window a cache of food hoarded by a local family - hams, butter, sugar, tins of various meats and all good things. The reason was unclear but perhaps it was to create some resentment - some had and some did not. If that was the purpose, it was a failure as no one I knew was resentful.

My main reason for being in this half square mile a lot during the first year was Billy Bunter. I used to collect a magazine called 'The Magnet' which featured Billy Bunter and Greyfriars School. The manager of Boots in Queen Street, a Mr Gould, collected these magazines for his son, Michael and we used to make swaps and loans. He lived in St. Brelade, he brought them to his office at Boots where I would visit to make the exchanges. Across from Boots is the Exeter pub where a school friend called Le Cocq lived. I would occasionally visit him. However the pearl in this oyster had to be West's Picture Palace which was located within this half square mile.

There were, of course, many times when rain or cold prevented outdoor excursions for we had neither raincoats nor overcoats fit to be seen. The only fires in the house would be the kitchen and sitting room, afternoons until bedtime. It was excessively cold in the bedrooms and on more than one winter's night a cup of water on the bedside table was a block of ice by the morning. But as our poet previously said - 'If winter comes, can Father Christmas be far behind?'

CHAPTER 7
PHANTOMS OF THE NIGHT

Both my hide-away and cache suffered major disruption in late 1943. The basement at Don Road had to be vacated as my parents moved to another property, also in Don Road. Whereas the first Don Road house was opposite Howard Davis Park, the second Don Road House was further up the hill and opposite Don Road Crescent. For ease of reference it shall be referred to as Don Road 2.

Fortunately the move was not at immediate notice and I had some days to empty the basement and transfer the contents to Don Road 2. This was achieved over five dark nights. My quandary was where to put all the objects I had collected for Don Road 2 had no unused basement.

The grenades were buried in a far corner of the garden, wrapped in a piece of canvas, the rifles, revolver, sword and ammunition were placed in a half roofed area of the garden shed, the tins of various foods, in a cupboard under books and magazines and under floor boards. With the exception of the food, which was depleted week by week, the rest were a real problem and remained so until Bob Cornish's garden became available to me.

Don Road 2 had one big advantage over Don Road 1. My bedroom was at the rear, on the first floor, with the bedroom window looking over the scullery roof. Therefore, it was easy to exit or enter my bedroom without being seen - over the scullery roof, through a side door in the garden wall and into Don Road.

Jock often used this route to visit me late at night, well after curfew. On his first appearance, woken by tapping at the window, I found Jock sitting on the scullery roof, waiting to be let in. I was astonished. Later, when he explained his route, I wondered at his bravery. Jock lived at Havre des Pas, little less than a mile from Don Road. His bravery was not that he had eluded German patrols, as we thought little of that, but he had come by way of Green Street Cemetery.

Green Street Cemetery was very old, largely unkempt and full of mausoleums, crosses, angels, trailing branches and overgrown paths. I had a fear of such places, possibly because my mother loved ghost stories and would often tell us of red eyed black horses with headless riders coming from or going to such places.

Jock took it in his stride, whereas I should much rather face a troop of S.S. led by Himmler himself, than go through Green Street Cemetery in the middle of the night. I once went through the Cemetery with Jock and held on to his coat tails for dear life and on another occasion, leaving him at Havre des Pas, I went home by the road - ghosts were much more frightening than Germans.

After Jock's first visit, he became a constant caller. Sometimes we just talked for an hour or two and at other times we went on the prowl. Our talks concerned Germans and raids, escape from Jersey and what to do after the war. We had no real ideas on that subject, mostly I must suppose because the normal progression from young boys to young men had been denied us. University or taking up a trade had been unavailable for years and we lived in the no-man's-land of waiting for the Germans to go. The present and its possibilities of excitement were our main concern.

We often went on the prowl as we found it easy to dodge German patrols. They were not numerous, but always about. We could hear them coming and even when they wore felt covers on their boots they talked and smoked. On hearing them, we could dodge up side streets or over garden fences or retreat until such hiding places were available. We wore dark clothes and soft shoes, holed and torn but very useful on our night prowls. We did not blacken our faces, although Jock, being dramatic and loving the parts we were playing, did suggest it. However, we had no blacking that could be easily removed and, if caught, could make up some story or other for being out after curfew but not very easily blackened faced: so reluctantly we discarded the idea.

We entered many German occupied hotels - for example, the grounds, garage and store of a hotel in Colomberie and the leisure area at the ground floor of a hotel in Green Street. We once went to the Grand Hotel which we entered easily enough through a ground floor window. The Germans had left the place some weeks earlier. It was quite eerie to roam the passageways, the smell of Germans strong in the air. In such a vast place, we stayed overlong and particular attention was needed to get home safely, particularly as our return route was through St.Helier.

One night we decided to visit our old favourite, the German clothing store near St Luke's school. We thought that the Germans might have added something or other to the store since our last visit.

The store was a dwelling house taken over by the Germans. It was an old house with servants quarters and with two entries - one to the main door up granite steps and the other, the servants entrance, down granite steps which curved, to place the servants door immediately below the main door. Both sets of steps were approached from the road pavement by way of an iron gate and short pathway.

Opposite the servants door, under the pathway and pavement was a coal-cellar. In the old days the coal-man would remove a circular iron manhole cover situated in the road pavement, tip his sacks of coal through this opening and fill the coal cellar. Our usual entry to this house was down the servants steps, around the house to the back and through a rear window.

On this particular night we had barely opened the iron gate when we heard a street patrol approaching. We rushed down the steps and stood quietly between the servants entrance door and the coal-house door. We heard the iron gate open and the two Germans footsteps on the pathway above. We were trapped! All we could do and did, was enter the coal-house. The door had no interior lock and our only security was to cling to the timber door with our fingernails to keep it shut. The silence of the coal-house was broken. Jock was at prayers, a loud Hail Mary full of grace. However, a hard elbow into his ribs and the prayers ceased.

Footsteps descended the granite steps and torch light gleamed through the edges of the coal house door as the Germans checked that the servants door was secure. The torch light went out, cigarettes were lit and a quiet conversation between the patrol guards continued for some minutes. Quiet as mice but with hearts pounding, we waited. Footsteps were heard on the steps and above us on the main door steps...faint rays of light as the security check was repeated...more footsteps descending the main steps, on the path. Then the iron gate squeaked open and clanged shut, footsteps in the road and they were gone.

We crept out of the coal-house, fingers numb with our efforts to keep the door tight. We could now both pray as loud as we wished. We had been within inches of two German guards, had got away with it and were very appreciative of our extreme good luck. We called it a day and both went home.

Jock and I had discussed an escape to France as, at this time in the story, the Allies had landed in France and had reached the French coast some 15 miles away from the north coast of Jersey. A year or two before I had worked for a market gardener, whose garden and sheds were in St Clements Inner Road. While working there, I had noticed two canvas canoes. They were dirty and littered with debris and appeared to be of little value to the owner. I asked the market gardener if he wanted them and, if not, could I have them? At first he said that they were of no use to him and I could have them but soon after changed his mind, for if I were caught with them he might well be in trouble.

To avoid any such mishap, he cut a square of canvas out of the bottom of each canoe and had workmen tie the canoes to rafters in the shed.

In my discussions with Jock I explained the possibility that these canoes were still hanging from the rafters in the very same shed. We could find canvas and repair them when our trip to France would be a real possibility. We decided to go in search of the canoes. We knew that it would take us a considerable time to walk to St Clement, get the canoes and haul them to Bob Cornish's garden, of which I now had the keys. We could not go before bed-time as we should be missed, so it had to be one of our late night escapades. So it was decided.

A few days after our discussion and final plan, Jock tapped at my window around midnight. We made good time to St.Clement, the market garden and the shed where all was silent and, with excited joy, found the canoes exactly where they should be. The canoes were cut down and taken from the shed with ease as they were not heavy but cumbersome. There were apples in the shed and we took two each to refresh us for the long haul to Bob Cornish's garden off Havre des Pas, a journey of less than three miles. We sat in silence and all around was silence, except for the crunch of bitten apples and an owl's hoot. Maybe we had disturbed him with our petty human concerns.

Apples finished, we started our journey with the canoes on either side of us, one in front and one behind, with left hands to the keels, fore and aft of one canoe and right hands in the same positions for the second canoe. This sounds easier than it was because our steps were uneven and our hands soon ached abominably. We tried carrying a canoe each, resting on our shoulders, our heads in the body of the canoe, the cockpit, or whatever it is called in respect to a canoe.

The canoes' prow had to be high in the air so that we could see where we were going. The wind often caught this sail-like surface and sent us staggering. We tried putting one canoe on top of the other but they were difficult to keep together and different muscles ached in response to the various methods used in carrying these burdens.

We had started off in high spirits but by halfway we were grumbling and bemoaning our task. A swear word or two was not uncommon and a certain amount of bickering occurred. Notwithstanding our troubles, we kept a keen watch for German patrols and hearing them coming we would, if possible, enter a side street, or dive over garden walls, the canoes thrown before us. The patrols were scarce and we had no real problems in that direction. Our two problems, inert and uncaring, were eventually brought to Bob Cornish's garden where we placed them in one of the sheds and hurried home, for it was now full light.

Jock lived a stones-throw away but I had a mile or more to go. Germans were now all over and it was impossible for me to dodge them but these were not patrols and, as I might well have been an early workman going to his place of work, they did not bother me. I arrived home sore and bruised but content, climbed over the scullery roof through the window, threw off filthy clothes and managed an hour's sleep before being called.

Although the worst was over, our canoe adventure had hardly started. We had to repair the canoes and to do that we had to find canvas and tar or bitumen. Bitumen was found under our noses. Jock's father had a drum in his garage, used for felt roof waterproofing. Canvas was another matter. We had to steal some and by steal do not mean from Germans as that would not be stealing. To steal in this case would be to take the canvas from someone or other of the local people.

Reprehensible as it was, we did just that. Jock had noticed some canvas awnings over the windows of a house in a cul -de- sac off the Havre des Pas road. We therefore, three nights after our collecting the canoes, slipped into the front garden of this house and, with a sharp knife, cut a large section out of one of the canvas awnings. I am sure that the lady who woke up in the morning to find a large hole in her sunshade would have forgiven us had she known of our need.

Everything ready, our ship building activities, unknown to Bob Cornish, could commence in Bob Cornish's shed. The work was soon carried out - the canoe canvas surfaces thoroughly brushed, bitumen applied to the existing canvas and the new canvas cut to size and dressed part way up the keel and up the side keel. Narrow strips of wood were tacked to both these keels to secure the canvas and a curved piece of timber covering the leading edge of the new canvas, all liberally covered with bitumen. We were ready to sail away!

We never did, for we were arrested in October and the canoes remained in the shed until after the war. When eventually used, they proved seaworthy. It was ironic that a house we had passed numerous times on both innocent and nefarious occasions was occupied by the Gestapo with whom we were soon to be forced to deal. The house was called Silvertide and we had once hidden among rocks almost under its windows when we had caused an explosion little more than one hundred and fifty yards away with complete disregard for the Gestapo as we were ignorant of their close proximity.

Of our exploits, our worst or best which ever way you see it, was to explode a German stick grenade. We had stick grenades in our possession and the desire to try one out became irresistible. Early one evening, just as the tide was level with the rear wall of the pool, we arrived there with a single stick grenade. Standing on the pool wall, we unscrewed the cap at the base of the stick, pulled on the toggle and threw the grenade into the sea.

We waited, but nothing happened. We were mystified but there was nothing to be done as the grenade was now ten feet under water, when we selected another grenade from our store we found that on screwing the head from the top of the grenade stick and closely examining both, we discovered a cylindrical aperture and it dawned on us that detonators were needed to explode the grenade. Further, we had such detonators among the bits and pieces we had picked up at German bunkers and at the time we had not known what they were. These were metal cylinders about an inch long and, when tried, fitted exactly the cylindrical void in the grenade. We selected another grenade and went back to the Pool a little after dusk on the following day when the tide would be suitable in being level with the Pool wall.

The grenade head was unscrewed from the stick, the detonator inserted, the grenade and stick screwed tightly back into position, we were ready. Strangely enough we had no misgivings, for our dealings with grenades was rudimentary and what was to follow was beyond our wildest imagination. The toggle was released from the base of the stick, pulled and the grenade thrown as far as possible into the sea. Seconds later, there was an underwater explosion, a great muffled roar and water blown high into the air. The pool wall shook and shuddered under our feet. We were at first aghast, then terrified, thinking that the whole German army would appear at any moment.

We ran around the pool wall, across the sand and hid among rocks which, unknown to us at the time, were just below and not more than twenty yards from Silvertide, the Gestapo Headquarters where in fear and trembling we waited. In the street above voices were heard, calling one to the other but this minor excitement soon died down and fifteen minutes later all was quiet.

We waited a little longer, crossed the beach and regained the road. It had been a most exciting experience but not one that we would try again. To calm and soothe our battered senses, we went to admire the canoes.

During our nights of roaming we had discovered a flour store and our last raid was to be on this German flour store one hundred yards down a cul-de-sac at Havre des Pas, almost opposite the Fort d'Auvergne Hotel. We carried out this raid just before curfew, the streets, as they

AUFRUF

AN DIE BEVOELKERUNG DER
INSEL JERSEY

Der Feind Deutschlands steht im Begriff, französischen Boden anzugreifen.

Ich erwarte von der Bevölkerung der Insel Jersey, dass sie unbedingt ruhig bleibt und auch bei Uebergreifen des Kampfes auf die Insel sich jeder feindlichen Haltung und Sabotage gegenüber der deutschen Wehrmacht enthält.

Bei Auftreten der geringsten Anzeichen von Unruhen werde ich die Strassen für jeden Verkehr sperren und Geiseln festnehmen lassen.

Angriffe auf die Wehrmacht werden mit dem Tode bestraft.

Der Kommandant der Festung Jersey,

HEINE,
Jersey, den 6. Juni 1944.   Oberst.

PROCLAMATION

TO THE POPULATION OF THE
ISLE OF JERSEY

Germany's enemy is on the point of attacking French soil.

I expect the population of Jersey to keep its head, to remain calm, and to refrain from any acts of sabotage and from hostile acts against the German Forces, even should the fighting spread to Jersey.

At the first signs of unrest or trouble I will close the streets to every traffic and will secure hostages.

Attacks against the German Forces will be punished by death.

Der Kommandant der Festung Jersey,

(Signed) HEINE,
Oberst.

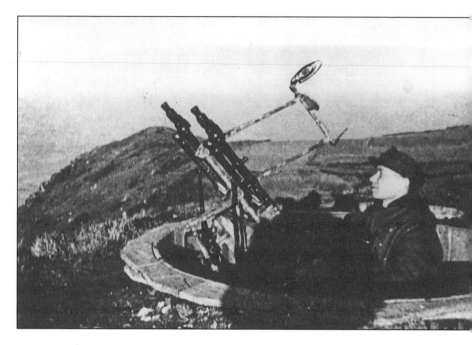

Above : D-Day Alert
Below : Silvertide, Gestapo Headquarters,
Havre des Pas

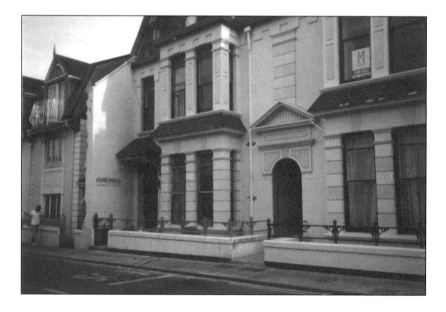

generally were, being empty of pedestrians and Germans alike. Except for German guards who patrolled La Collette to the Middle Rock at Greve d'Azette, we had little to fear.

We watched these guards pass on their way to Greve d'Azette and as soon as they were well away, approached the flour store. The door was of a simple timber construction with the usual padlock and within two minutes we were inside. The store was filled with stacks of 50kg bags of flour. We found a porter's type trolley, loaded a sack and set off down Havre des Pas to Jock's house some two hundred yards away.

The trolley made the most awful noise, the wheels screeching for want of oil. We wanted to run with the trolley but when we did, the screeching reached a crescendo. Screams and wails filled the street and listeners cowering behind closed doors must have thought that banshees were abroad that night or the Germans were up to no good with the thumbscrew.

We arrived at the yard door where Jock's father met us. How he knew we were about our Occupation trade I do not know but he had certainly heard us for he had an oil can in his hand and thoroughly oiled the trolley wheels. We then returned for more flour and ran two and fro with a total of four sacks. the trolley behaving sweetly with a gentle rumble of its wheels on the tarmac.

We replaced the trolley and secured the store door. Our raid may not have been noticed as there were hundreds of sacks of flour and four would not be missed. Also the damaged door might well be due to rough handling by workmen. I went home with one sack but, in four journeys over the next four days. Jock's father was to give two sacks away to needy families.

Perhaps because we had suffered two major scares or because the water polo was reaching its end of season series of matches, the 'Phantoms of the Night' retired.

CHAPTER 8
THE GARDEN

The garden was located between Green Street and Roseville Street, approached by way of Green Street by means of a short lane leading to high granite walls and a three feet by seven feet single door built into the wall or by way of Havre des Pas by means of a longish lane leading to another granite wall with a double gate for vehicular traffic - Bob's horse and cart. It was no Garden of Eden but it might be considered a 'Secret Garden' as both approach lanes led to other similar walled areas and the two entrances were incidental to the many other, better maintained gates and doorways.

The garden area was approximately two acres, entirely surrounded by high granite walls and subdivided into three land parcels by similar granite walls. These interior walls were partly demolished in places to allow access from one parcel to the other. Ferns and various flora sprouted from the cracks and crannies in the walls. The most prolific was a green leafed, long stemmed red flower.

Mr Day, a florist, owned a similar garden on the Roseville Street side of this half square mile of gardens. His shop was in Bath Street immediately opposite West's cinema. When flowers were in short supply, Mr Day would fill the shop windows with these red flowers, not for sale, but to show that his business continued. He would place the red flowers on white shelves interspersed with blue flowerpots. Such was Mr Day's simple act of defiance.

This type of property was common in the area bordering Green Street and Roseville Street and the original purpose always puzzled me, for there were no houses within them and it was difficult to understand why anyone would construct a series of high walled enclosures coming from and going nowhere.

However, for privacy and for my purpose, Bob's garden was invaluable.

The landlord, Bob Cornish, was a man of thirty or so, medium height, dark hair, of heavy build and quiet and unassuming. He played water polo for the Beeches Old Boys and therefore I knew him well and on my leaving the Beeches in July 1944, he offered me the job of looking after his garden and I was happy to accept. We both agreed that it would keep me gainfully employed until the end of the Occupation until Christmas. We were both wrong. The Occupation lasted another nine months and I lasted in the garden for less than three months.

Bob's father was a farmer with a farm in St Saviour and whether or not the garden was owned or leased by Bob or his father, I never did find out. However, Bob was in charge. I had no connection with the farm and visited it two or three times at the most, met his father once but never met his mother or two of his three sisters. One sister I did meet was Dora, a blond buxom lady a little older than Bob. I was seldom in her company - once at the farm and on odd occasions when she visited the garden with Bob. She fascinated me to such an extent that when she spoke to me I blushed, trembled and was tongue tied. This amused her, for on such occasions she laughed and waggled away. She was exotic and full of mellow fruitfulness and I must owe my first sexual twinge to Dora.

The garden, in reality a vegetable plot, was planted with carrots, beans, onions, turnips, potatoes and sweetcorn. Sweetcorn was the main crop and covered seventy-five per cent of the arable land. Picking sweetcorn was my main occupation for the first few weeks. The cobs were picked and placed into boxes which Bob and his horse and cart would collect twice weekly together with two or three boxes of other vegetables.

Except for a two day stint when Bob and I went through the whole sweetcorn plantation picking the few remaining cobs, Bob's visits to the garden became once each week. I was entirely on my own except for his vegetable collection or 'See how things are going' days. Within reason my working hours were my own to choose -always provided the work was done. I always finished by 4pm then off to the Pool, little more than two hundred yards down Havre des Pas.

The privacy and remoteness of the garden, caused by the high granite walls - although variable in height but never less than twenty feet - was a godsend to me. I was now able to remove all my German trophies from Don Road. Careless youth gave little thought to Bob Cornish and family. It was most likely disloyal but I was in a quandary.

Bob's susceptibilities were to be sorely tried by the Gestapo's expatiation of his many sins and the ungrateful child. The serpents bite would be secondary. I, of course, thought of none of this and moved my trophies to the garden in high glee. In very small loads and night by night I removed everything from Don Road to Bob's garden.

Rifles, ammunition, revolver, machine gun barrels and uniforms were all stored in one of the many dilapidated sheds in the garden. My German officer's sword I had recently acquired was placed in the tool shed for I had thought of an excellent use for it. The hand grenades were dug up from the Don Road garden and re-buried more safely in the upper reaches of Bob's garden.

At the foot of a wall, immediately adjacent to its foundations, I dug a hole four feet deep, placed both the pineapple grenades and the stick grenades in the bottom, covered them with granite wall blocks obtained from the demolished part of an interior wall. I filled the remaining three feet with soil and replaced the sods of grass, wild flowers and weeds that I had carefully removed and put aside. Within a week or two it was impossible to notice any difference between the adjoining area and the grenade pit and two months later I had no idea where the pit was.

At the end of the Occupation I told a British Intelligence sergeant of the grenades somewhere along the foot of the wall. He said that German prisoners would dig until they located them. Whether this was done or not I do not know. I now had the weapons and ammunition and I also had a place to fire them. Thursdays was German practice day.

In sympathy, Thursday became my practice day. Waiting until the sound of gunfire could be heard round and about, I set up my targets and fired at will with both the rifle and the revolver. I only had six or so lead bullets for the revolver. I used two but was reluctant to use them all. However, I discovered that the rifle bullets fitted the revolver, or rather the cartridge case did, the detonator head fitting exactly into the revolver chamber. The bullet was smaller than the revolver barrel and when the revolver was fired, the bullet left the barrel turning over and over. This was evidenced by the elongated holes in the timber I fired at. The cartridge case and bullet were longer than the revolving chamber and therefore could not revolve on firing and only one shot at a time was possible.

The rifle, on the other hand, fired its five shots as quickly as I could withdraw and ram home the bolt. The machine gun bullets fitted the rifle. They were exactly the same size and, taking them off the belt, they could be used as rifle bullets. By this means a puzzle was solved as every fifth bullet on the machine gun belt was tipped with black or white. The black were armour piercing, the white were tracers. The black went through very heavy bulks of timber to flatten themselves on the granite wall behind, the white caught the timber alight.

This was a nine day wonder for me and on my first days practice I over indulged. Mine was the last practice to finish. The novelty wore off and except for an odd shot with the revolver which with a few rifle bullets were easily hidden conveniently to hand, the rifle and ammunition were hidden and forgotten. The rifle was thoroughly cleaned and oiled, including the barrel, for I had a cleaning brush - a cylindrical brush with a long chain. The chain was dropped down the barrel to appear at the other end, pulled through dragging the brush through the barrel. Usually the chain was passed through the bolt end for, as the brush came through the barrel, it turned, following and cleaning the rifling.

My work was easy and often friends called and would share a mug of soup. In one of the more out of the way, dilapidated sheds, I had built a fireplace by the use of bricks and a steel drain cover. I obtained an old saucepan and was able to fill this with vegetables, boil them for some time and a good vegetable soup resulted.

The fireplace was built where it was unlikely to be noticed by Bob and the vegetables used were often bruised and damaged, not fit for the market but with rotten and bruised segments cut out, they were perfectly good for soup. There were onions, cabbages, beans, carrots and potatoes improved by the addition of crushed sweetcorn. It was very good soup and I received many compliments on my cooking, even if both the weather and the soup were hot.

We also made dandelion coffee. This was made from the roots of the dandelion plant, washed and roasted on the grill, crushed to a powder and instant coffee was available. It was bitter but not too unlike coffee. Insofar as real coffee had no great attraction for us, this dandelion coffee had none at all. However, it was fun to make. Older people were always searching for substitutes for tea and coffee. Roasted acorns, parsnips, wheat and much else were the cause of experiments. Soup kitchens, run by the States of Jersey, were located in the town and often used the Chelsea Hotel soup kitchen in Gloucester Street. However, with the plentiful supply of waste vegetables my soup kitchen became popular.

The Indian corn - sweetcorn - was finished. All the cobs had been picked and it only remained to cut the stalks and remove them so that the ground could be ploughed and prepared for the early potato planting. It was my job to cut the stalks which was likely to be long, hard work as many were two inches in diameter and six to seven feet tall. The German officer's sword had come to mind and I would turn the work of cutting into a game.

There was an old fashioned circular grinding wheel in one of the sheds. The grinding wheel with a steel turning handle was mounted on a wooden frame with a water trough within which the bottom section of the wheel rotated. When the trough was filled with water the grindstone was constantly wet as it was rotated. To sharpen the sword the handle was turned round and round, keeping the sword blade pressed to the grindstone. For ease of use and a keen edge this required two people but I managed and the sword soon had a fine edge.

The sword, without its scabbard, had been obtained from German officer's quarters at the Beaufort Hotel. The scabbard was most likely in the same room but not immediately to be seen on quick entry and exit through an open window. It was a fine weapon of polished steel with gold filigree at the hilt. I never knew the rank or titles of its owner.

With drawn sword, glittering in the sunlight, I advanced to do battle. The enemy was waiting, rank upon rank, ten thousand strong, column upon menacing column, taller than me and prepared for battle. With drawn sword, I attacked their first line of defence, highly trained S.S. men who fought with grim determination and no quarter given or asked. The bugle sounded truce from time to time as my trusty sword required to be sharpened and I needed a drink and a bucket of water poured over my head.

This was shortly to be improved upon as the heat and perspiration generated by my struggles was oppressive. I filled a water butt with water, stripped down and jumped in where I would stay for three or four minutes, returning to do battle in just my underpants and shoes. By four o'clock of that first day, the bugles sounded truce when the S.S. were in a state of utter defeat. The victor saluted the fallen and went to the Pool for a swim.

The next morning, very early to catch the enemy by surprise, I attacked the Goths. Brave fighters as they were, they fell under my strong arm and trusty sword. Insofar as my trusty sword needed sharpening, the whetstone was necessary for every five hundred enemy slain and I needed a drink and a water butt bath. There were many truces. The Duke of Burgundy's men were soon conquered and when at bugle time at 4pm the second day, only Attila the Hun and some of Dora's admirers loitering to the rear, were left for the following day.

Attila and his mounted horsemen were a fearful band but with slashing, cutting, hacking and with blood curling yells and screams, louder and more frightening than all Attila's hoard, they were overcome. By the afternoon's jump in the water barrel, ignominious defeat was theirs. They had fought well, for my trusty sword had to be sharpened nine times and there was very little left to sharpen.

The remainder, Dora's admirers, fell twenty minutes later. It took time as Dora had a lot of admirers - a sorry bunch when compared with my previous adversaries. The big, good-looking, dark haired admirer was beheaded, then felled. It was finished! Ten thousand had sunk to the ground overpowered, the weary to sleep and the wounded to die. Bob's cornfield was cleared. The conqueror, the weary one, swaggered to the Pool.

When the Gestapo found the German officers sword, saw its condition and became aware of the use it had been put to, they were more upset by this single misdemeanour than all the others I had committed; notwithstanding their anger it had served a better purpose than it had ever done in the past, i.e. saluting Hitler!

Bob was amazed when he arrived and found the whole field of corn had been cut. He had come to help with the cutting but instead he helped load the corn stalks on to his horse drawn wagon and that was our occupation for a further three days. The corn stalks, once loaded, were taken to a corner of the field and dumped. By chance the dump was very close to the grenade pit and Neddy, the horse with whom I was in a constant state of war, pricked up his ears when he heard me mutter 'Come on Neddy, you fat bellied excuse for a nightmare, a little closer and blow yourself to horses heaven.'

I understand that Neddy was named after a Jersey States member called 'Ned' who had helped Mr Cornish in Neddy's purchase. I was to blame for our state of war as I had teased Neddy on the first day I saw him. I was in the barn loft when Bob drove him in and stopped Neddy just inside the barn entrance and immediately under my feet. I had tied a carrot to a piece of string and lowered it just in front of his nose. He lifted his head to take a bite and I quickly pulled the carrot up and away. This happened three or four times until, with his head high in the air, he saw me, I laughed at him and he stamped and snorted. I had made an enemy. I tried to make friends for on coming down from the loft I had tried to give him the carrot but he sulked and would have nothing to do with me.

His revenge came quickly, for within a day or two as I was squeezing past him where he stood in the barn entrance, he shuffled over and trapped me in the corner made by the wall and the barn door-frame. I pushed at him as hard as I could but he pushed back and easily won the trial of strength. Pleading and threatening made no difference and I stayed his prisoner for ten minutes or more until Bob came to my rescue. I had used my one trick but Neddy had many, he nipped me, nudged me and snorted when close enough to make me jump. It took many carrots to mollify him but we were friends in the end.

It became more than ever obvious that the war would soon be over and with it the Occupation. Heavy gunfire was a daily occurrence coming from France - across the water some fifteen miles away. Planes were continuously passing overhead, British or American, on their way to France and Germany. The German anti-aircraft guns often fired but more as a show of spite rather than for any real objective or hope of hitting anything.

The German forces became more numerous by the addition of troops being evacuated from France and brought to Jersey. These were units that had been surrounded by the Allies in the St Malo area and Jersey was their only means of escape. They were mainly shabby, tired and hungry although many of the old guard remained, the nucleus to put the backbone in the coming battle that was expected.

The aeroplanes and the gunfire from France lessened and ceased altogether. The Allies had finished their work in our area and we were once again abandoned. In retrospect this was the only sensible thing to do as the Island was a fortress and any attack would have resulted in heavy casualties for attacker, defender and the local population. However, it was sad to be left for a further eight months.

The Germans, with so many troops and nothing to do, increased their patrols and most stores and gun bunkers were guarded twenty four hours each day. Our gun bunker in Green Street was under permanent guard. This must have been due to the Germans expecting an attack at any time, an attack which never materialised.

Wars could be forgotten at the pool. During August and September 1944 the water polo matches were at their height. Working at the garden gave me plenty of freedom to visit the pool daily. To ensure this, I started very early and could always leave the garden, three hundred yards from the pool, at 4pm. Isolated from the Germans, wars and normal life itself, I swam, practiced and played. We, of course, discussed the end of the war but what this would mean and what we should do was beyond our comprehension.

From the pool, looking north-east and some two hundred yards away, the goddess of retribution waited, the storms clouds were gathering and the Gestapo of Silvertide were soon to pounce. Happily, of this I was blissfully unaware.

CHAPTER 9
ARREST

The Gestapo, led by Herr Karl accompanied by three of his merry men, arrived at Don Road No. 2 in the early evening of a dark October night in 1944. They knocked, demanded entry and entered without any polite preamble - almost music hall characters in their long coats or raincoats, black dominating and all wearing slouch hats which they failed to remove. They jostled their way through the hallway and through the first open doorway which proved to be the sitting room, named in vain for this visit as they made no move to sit down.

This was not a social call and serious business of the Third Reich was to be accomplished. They demanded to see me who, standing three feet away from them, put my hand up, my vocal chords being rather restricted. Herr Karl said little more than that he was taking me with him and two men would stay to search the house. I was taken away by Karl and his mate, two being left behind to carry out the search and my family left in fear and trembling. I, myself, was by no means carefree but I was mystified. I had not been caught doing anything that the Germans might frown upon and, in that direction, I had been as good as gold for five or six weeks. We had lived dangerously for four years, our only safeguard being never to be caught. Wits, fleetness of foot and punch-ups had been used to this end.

At the eleventh hour (and it was the eleventh hour as France had been liberated) the Germans surrounded and isolated in the Channel Isles, our luck had run out. It was time to pay the piper! Karl pushed me into the back seat of a black limousine standing at the curbside, climbed in beside me and his minion - proven to be so by shouted orders of Karl. The driver took us around the corner, down St.Clement's Road, a right turn and there was Gestapo Headquarters, Silvertide!

Silvertide stood and still stands at the east end of Havre des Pas, just before the Greve D'Azette end of Havre des Pas. It is the first of two exactly similar houses and borders the sea. We all entered and I was taken to the first room on the right which proved to be the sitting or drawing room, perhaps the former for the house was not all that grand. I was sat at a table, where I sat for nigh on three hours in silence and alone. There was a guard posted near the door, sitting on a chair in the hallway. This I discovered when I decided that a visit to the toilet was necessary and also would break the monotony.

When I opened the door in search of a toilet the guard jumped up, violently pushed me back into the room and stood in the doorway shouting questions. He spoke very little English, so with hissing noises and hand gestures to suit, I made my needs known. It seemed that he did not have the authority to deal with the calls of nature, could not leave the hallway and was calling, rather hesitatingly, for assistance.

Someone arrived, for I heard a brief conversation, silence, then some other, presumably a more senior Gestapo man arrived. I wondered if they had to call Hitler to obtain permission for me to pee? Ten minutes from my first request and after much leg crossing and uncrossing, hops and jumps, I was taken by the hall guard to a toilet further down the passage. He held me tightly by the arm going, kept the toilet door open with his foot, watched all my movements and gripped me firmly by the arm on the way back.

I was a little proud for I thought that they would not have taken better care of Mr Churchill had he been their prisoner. I also became fearful for they were taking prodigious care of me. Just as I was thinking of another telephone call to Mr Hitler, the reason for the long delay in the expected interrogation was explained. Karl, a more senior Gestapo man called Wolf or Wolfgang and a third (an observer?) for he said nothing all night and, during the interrogation, came and went as he saw fit.

They had found little or nothing at the house, a few cans and packets of food, armbands, all with swastikas, German first aid kits, bits and pieces and a packet of opium. The opium had come from the Merton Hotel and, I supposed, used as a painkiller. I, in my various Boys Own magazines, had read of cunning Chinese planning some treacherous deed or other, smoking opium. I had left the opium in the house thinking that one day I would find a Chinese pipe, smoke and dream multicoloured dreams and not multicoloured nightmares which was now my lot. I was lost! The Gestapo, finding little at the house, had asked my parents where I worked and they, in all innocence, had given Bob Cornish's name.

In some German way or another, they had located the farm at St Saviour and, on being informed that I worked at the garden at Havre des Pas less than a half mile from Silvertide, they had forced Bob Cornish to go with them to the garden and had carried out a preliminary search. With the aid of torches and less than an hour's search, they had found enough for their night's entertainment to begin.

We sat at a round table, Karl, Wolf and the unknown on one side and I sat across from them, my back to the door. A reading lamp had been placed on the table, swivelled so that more light shone on me than on them. Their shoulders down to their arms and hands could be seen but their faces were in shadow, whereas mine was fully in the light. The lamp was not too bright and its light on my face was not either intimidating or greatly uncomfortable.

They had found the rifle and ammunition hidden in the loft of the main barn and told me that a full search would be made in the morning. They, of course, asked how I came to possess a German soldier's rifle and ammunition. 'I found it on the back of a lorry' was no good and Wolf slapped the table hard when I suggested my forlorn hope. The slapping of the table was their response when they were angry. I told them that I had stolen it from the Merton Hotel armoury over a year ago. With whom? What other German facilities had I and my friends robbed? They were well informed concerning many of our raids and their information was unlikely to have come from an anonymous letter.

I came to understand that I was not the first to be questioned. I was later to see how their arrests and questioning had produced a domino effect. The first raider caught (and I was never to know who he might be) had, in toppling, led to the next who, in his turn, toppled and so to my turn. I must suppose that I toppled for they questioned me for most of the night. They were professionals and I was soon to become a witless tool in their hands. As most of my friends had been arrested before me, I was later to take comfort that someone had pulled the plug and we were all in the whirlpool, most likely because of the one, or ones, first caught in some raid or other.

Their interest was intense with regard to the ringleader and I had been cast in that role. Who were my contacts? To whom did I report? Bemused, I became aware that they were certain that there was an adult organisation by whom we or I had been guided, that the weapons and arms discovered were less than had been stolen from the German forces. I thought this unlikely as it must be doubted that all the arms we had taken into our possession would have been reported and listed.

They were right with respect to thirty or so bullets, missing a crate of pineapple grenades and a half dozen stick grenades. The bullets may have been counted by the number of bullet holes in three or four timber targets in Bob Cornish's garden. The grenades were never found and the Gestapo were to remain ignorant of the existence of these deadly weapons. They were also to remain in ignorance of the cause of the explosion some three months before, less than three hundred yards from their beds.

The questioning, from tack to tack, always returned to an underground organisation waiting to move when Jersey was invaded by the Allied Forces. They believed it inconceivable that Britain would ignore the Channel Isles with troops little more than twenty miles away.

They did not hit or beat me, the table was the recipient of their anger. They served coffee from time to time and I was to find my only friend, in that friendless house, in the person who served the coffee.

He was also the only person in uniform - an oldish soldier with an exaggerated limp. His walk was a deliberate one step at a time movement and, either by necessity or nature, completely unhurried. His coffee serving could last ten minutes but without reprimand from my fellow guests for coffee. I wondered if the coffee was mine for I had concealed two packets under my bedroom floorboards. If so, they were in truth my guests.

This old soldier, when carefully placing the coffee before me, always gave me a smile and placed his hand on my shoulder when his hand was free of the cup. He paid no attention to his superiors in doing this, all that could be done to him had been done, he had no fear for anything worse. Whether his smile and touch were a token of pity or encouragement, I did not know. I think the latter, whatever, it was comforting. I mentioned him to the British when they released me from prison seven months later. They told me that they would quickly repatriate known good Germans. I hope that he went home to some comfort for he was certainly the best German I have ever known.

Questioning continued but near dawn, tired of their own questions they called it a day, almost satisfied that there was no underground organisation. However, Karl, his great coup in ruins, retained lingering hopes of running to earth the Jersey underground army. It was foolish in the extreme to imagine an armed resistance movement. The Island was little more than seventy square miles with neither mountains nor forests. Resistance of the passive variety was almost total and was remarkable in its uncoordinated longevity. Germans did not exist with respect to either common courtesy or social contact. A German officer of the Command Headquarters bitterly complained to a Jersey States Minister, that 'We are ghosts in this Country.'

They took me home at 5.30am where I found my mother, red eyed and distraught, sitting waiting. She quickly rose and started to make up the remaining embers of the fire, saying that she would make me some porridge. Karl did not interfere but when I noticed my mother putting green wood onto the embers, I left the room, to be followed by Karl. I went to the garden shed and collected an armful of dry wood and was returning to the house when Karl called me to a patch of ground which he was staring at intently.

He had found the filled-in hole where the grenades had once been buried. We went back into the house and whilst I was making up the fire, Karl called to the car driver, sitting in his parked car. The driver came in and Karl indicated that he should wait until I had the fire burning brightly. He then asked me to go with him and the driver into the garden. A spade was found in the garden shed and Karl set the driver to work, digging in the disturbed ground area. The driver worked with gusto and ten minutes later was digging into hard packed earth. Karl lost interest and we returned indoors.

Some watery but good porridge was ready and Mother, always the lady, treated the Gestapo like - unwanted but by necessity - guests. The whole family had arrived by now and questions and answers were thrown to and fro to which Karl made no objection. I did my best to comfort my mother by telling her that all my friends were in prison and that we were sure to enjoy ourselves! Whatever Karl thought of that he kept to himself but being German he most likely thought I meant what I said and pondered over the apparent eccentricities of the British. With hugs all round, I was taken to the German prison.

The German prison was in two separate blocks of cells forming part of the Jersey prison in Gloucester Street. However, it was completely separated and formed no part of the Jersey prison and was administered and run by uniformed Germans. By some blunder on the part of the guard to whom I was entrusted by Karl, I was put in a cell occupied by Don. After initial suspicious riposte and parry, we realised that neither of us were the first one in the domino collapse. We discussed our situation and soon gloomily agreed that the Gestapo knew almost everything there was to know and we were in serious trouble. Don was taken away within an hour of my arrival, the guard having realised his error and three hours later Karl and the Gestapo driver took me away for a visit to Bob Cornish's garden.

When we arrived, a thorough search was underway. Six uniformed soldiers were helping three plain clothed Gestapo men. Bob Cornish was also there and was not very pleased with me. The search uncovered everything hidden there with the exception of the grenades, although they did find a box of detonators. They, of course found the canoes but strangely enough paid little attention to them. Numerous questions arose when they could not match the various items discovered and Karl's list was a series of ticks and question marks:

Rifle and rifle bullets
Machine gun bullets, no gun?
Revolver and revolver bullets
Pistol bullets, no pistol?
Grenade detonators, no grenades?
Two machine gun barrels??
Two bayonets?

The many miscellaneous items were listed without comment. I knew of this list and its ticks and question marks as, when they had exhausted their search, Karl indicated a wooden trestle and we both perched on its three inch support beam. His list was in German but he read out the objects one by one and questioned me on the, in his opinion, missing items. I convinced him that I was merely a collector and took most objects out of interest. Rifles and bullets had been easy to find, as had machine gun bullets but machine guns, owing to their size and weight, were impossible.

The pistol bullets had been found but I had never found a pistol. 'Why the machine gun barrels?' Karl asked. Because they were perfect collectors items in themselves, works of art in their precise engineering. Karl was pleased with the reply and was eloquent in his praise of German engineering. The detonators raised a single question only and my reply that they had been collected without my knowing what they were for, satisfied Karl. Our tête-a-tête was ended by shouts and curses from the erstwhile searchers, the sword had been found.

The German officer's sword had been placed against the barn wall with other tools and had not been discovered until that moment. Brought into the full light, it was a pitiful object - the fretwork of the hilt bent and twisted, a mere half inch width of blade remaining and six inches missing from the end. I described its use whilst in my possession, the corn had to be cut and I was heavily cuffed by one of the Gestapo. Karl yelled at him just in time, for another blow was coming and I was more than ready to give better than I received. The cuff had been hard and unexpected and anger had driven all the restraint from my mind.

Bob was called over. The exchange had unnerved him and he was pale and hesitant when he approached. Poor Bob! All the blame was heaped upon his head - it was his garden, he was the boss, why did he let it happen? All his replies and excuses were ignored and he received a ten minute harangue of insults. All were allowed to participate and Bob was soon drowning in a sea of scorn and ridicule. Most of this was in German but the intent was clear enough.

As for me, I was the innocent bystander giving Neddy a wink from time to time. As for Neddy, Bob's only transport to the garden, I could see his big green teeth exposed and ready. I was in hope that a German would get too close to him when an arm or shoulder would get an awful bite. It did not happen and in this Bob was lucky for if he could not be expected to entirely control his farm boy, he would be completely responsible for the control of his horse!

Knowing Neddy, I was certain that Bob was not in full control. In all these exchanges and for a time I thought that they might arrest

Bob and let me go, I wondered if any thought was given to the owner of the sword? Poor fellow, he was in all likelihood, long since dead in the Russian snow.

Pats and good-byes to Neddy, who gazed at me sadly, a 'never mind' to Bob who gazed at me with some resentment. Hello prison!

CHAPTER 10
PRISON

My new home was to be the German prison which was located within the overall complex of the Jersey prison on Gloucester Street in St Helier. The main entrance served both the local and German prisons. Enter this gate, tended by local guards, up a concrete footpath in a gravel yard area and straight ahead this was the local prison. Turn an abrupt left, just before reaching the local prison entrance gates along another path between high granite walls the German prison steel door entrance was located.

All these areas were surrounded by high granite walls, thirty feet high on the Gloucester Street and Newgate Street sides and mostly twenty five feet in height separating the German prison from the local prison.

The German section was in two parts. On its northern flank a two storied cell block containing forty cells, twenty to each floor and populated by British prisoners, the southern flank, a similar building but much older, for German wrongdoers, deserters and the like. Between these two cell blocks were the exercise yards, guards quarters, kitchens and ablutions. The whole, damp, dark and forbidding.

I was taken to a cell in the British block and lodged on the first floor in a cell at the end of the corridor. The cell was approximately ten by twelve feet with stone walls and a small, arched steel-grilled window. The door was of steel with a peephole but no keyhole on the inside. It was locked by snap locks and, when pushed closed, the lock tongues snapped into the locked position. The furniture consisted of a low level bed constructed of plywood, six inches off the floor, a boxed plywood headrest. The mattress was of dirty, heavy cloth stuffed with straw. There was one shabby, not too clean blanket. A cracked chamber pot stood in one corner. There was nothing else in the cell.

On being pushed into this cell, the door slammed shut with the snap of the lock tongues locked in position and the overriding thought was how to get out of this cage. Escape ideas came and remained foremost in my mind. I was to remain in this cell alone for six weeks. I had visits from Karl which were welcome for they relieved the monotony and as I had nothing more to say other than repeat what I had previously said, we would often discuss unconnected subjects.

However, his visits soon stopped and except for exercise periods, two each day lasting, in all, one hour I spent twenty three hours each day alone, which was a price to be paid and I had no real regrets. Karl, during my first interrogation at Gestapo Headquarters did ask me if I was sorry and ashamed at what I had done. I, of course, said yes but in fact I was as sorry as a frog may be expected to be and less ashamed than Hitler's teddy bear.

The food was served in the cell thee times daily, a mug of something called coffee and a lump of bread in the morning and a mug of soup and another lump of bread at midday and evening. The soup was almost always cabbage with disgusting pieces of meat floating on the surface, pallid white, most likely intestines. Once in spooning out a solid piece from the bottom of the mug, I picked out a small piece of jawbone with a greenish black tooth still imbedded in the bone.

Soup was over for that day. However, needs must and thereafter I spooned out the floating pieces into the chamber pot and never went near the bottom of the mug. The chamber pots were emptied and washed by the prisoners on their way to and from exercise.

Books were a luxury but from time to time I obtained one from kind fellow prisoners. I once read A Child's Introduction to Shakespeare three or four times with great relish. Six weeks over, I moved into the company of the living. I was moved to another cell and joined two other prisoners. One was a youth called Bill Bennett and he was to help me in my first escape attempt, some weeks later.

Our particular guards were three in number:, Otto, Heinrich and the Chief, Cheffy or Swinehault. Otto was a short, fat man, pot bellied and with a Punch shaped nose with all sorts of bumps and swellings. He was stupid and a bully, always yelling 'Los Los,' 'Snell Snell,' 'Hahen Hahen' and such other shouts and yells to maintain his authority. He was also a coward, for on one occasion he yelled at the top of his voice inches from my head, I turned on him and made a charade of wringing his scrawny neck and he backed quickly away, fear spread over his face. Nothing came of it but he kept his distance thereafter.

Heinrich, a tall, slender man of regular features, was quiet and watchful. There was an undercurrent of dissatisfaction and anger in his whole being. The rise of the Third Reich had been unkind, for he had no rank and its impending fall was the unkindest cut of all. He should have been happy with his present, danger free occupation but he was dangerous and needed to be watched.

Cheffy, pronounced Heffy, was similar in appearance to Otto but with no bumps to his nose. His rank was obscure - some sort of Warrant Officer as he wore no stripes. He ordered and instructed and strutted. Nothing was better in his life than Heil Hitler-ing Karl or another of Karl's gang when they appeared at the prison. At that late date Cheffy was still in pursuit of the Iron Cross! Other than shouting his orders in a very loud voice, mostly to his subordinates, he was no cause for concern and was, in the main, ignored.

This prison was a miserable place, damp, cold and dirty. The guards, having been told that they were the *Master Race* for a large part of their lives and, having no ideas how to act the part, were cold, dead men despite occasional attempts at jovial Uncle Fritz. Bullies all and shouting orders or shouting for no reason whatsoever but to show that they were in command was their daily bread. Worst of all, they were stupid as they might have carried out their duties in a more relaxed, humane manner but they had no inbred knowledge of kindness or humility when dealing with lesser souls.

I was much later to be a prisoner in Iraq and during that period I compared the Iraqi guards with the German guards of the Occupation. The Iraqi guards were superior men, their duty was to guard, not to bully and bluster. When it was within their power, they made life easier with smiles and a joy of life, notwithstanding that they lived under the rule of a similar dictatorship. I am not saying that they would not shoot you if ordered to do so but they would do it with regret.

As an example, during my hostage days in Iraq exercise was confined to a yard area, not dissimilar to our German prison yard though rather larger in area. To break the monotony of walking around and around during exercise, I would kick a football. The Iraqi guards had erected a net at one corner of the yard where they played handball, using the football. It often happened that when I appeared in the yard for my walk, the guards were playing handball. They always stopped the game, saying 'Here is your ball, Mr. Richard!' and they would throw the ball to me. Otto, Heinrich and Cheffy were unlikely to play handball and most unlikely to hand over the ball if they did.

In the German prison suffering was not uncommon and was felt by many of its inmates. To a few suffering was intense and moans and groans of restless sleepers and sometimes sobbing could be heard in the night. I suppose that we were all responsible for our plight but the sobs were of mental pain not of remorse. I was fine, for I had much to do - the game remained afoot.

My first plan of escape was executed in early December. Jock was imprisoned in the local prison area, as just before his arrest he had injured his eye in taking a gun spring bolt to pieces and the spring had fired the pin into his eye. He was receiving almost daily medical treatment at the General Hospital, the next building to the prison. From time to time I received messages from Jock although I could not return any answer. The local prison, being on a higher level or of extra height, notes could be tossed over the wall during our exercise period.

Jock proposed that if I could by some means, get to the hospital any Monday, Wednesday or Friday, we could meet and make our escape. There was only one way to get to the hospital and that was an injury that needed immediate attention. Bill Bennet agreed to cut my arm open. To make it look like an accident, I was to put on a shirt much too big for me, with the sleeves way below my hands and in cutting the arms of the shirt to a reasonable length, the razor blade had cut into my arm. So it was planned and so it worked. The shirt on, Bill cut part way through the sleeve, asked if I was ready and, at a nod, cut into my arm just below the elbow. It was a surgeon's job, a deep cut, plenty of blood and acceptable as an accident, I still have the scar to this day.

Shouting and hammering at the doors brought Otto to the scene where, seeing blood, he dashed out in panic and returned with both Cheffy and Heinrich. He had left the cell door open when he dashed away. The memory of this incident was to remain in my mind, although without particular importance at the time, it was to resurface and be of use at a later date.

Unfortunately Heinrich, the most alert of all the guards, escorted me to the hospital. We walked the short distance to the outpatients department, the torn off sleeve acting as a bandage. We passed the Chelsea Hotel where the States of Jersey ran a soup kitchen. I had used it and the soup served was decidedly better than the prison soup. On arrival at the hospital, the nurses, not knowing of my ulterior motive, acted with great kindness and expedition, whereas I wished to hang about and weigh up the situation. There was no sign of Jock.

Two nurses led me to the surgery of the out-patients department and glared at Heinrich when he insisted on accompanying us. They sat me down, one cleaned the wound whilst the other prepared needle and thread. The nurses asked questions and a conversation of prison and of a more trivial nature followed. Trivial because I was anxious to know where Jock was. I slipped this question in during our talk and was told that he was always taken to a private room down the corridor where he then was with his parents.

During most of this conversation Heinrich called for silence, which requests were ignored. The needle came into play and I received four or five stitches. When that was over and despite Heinrich's protests, the nurses insisted that I sit for ten minutes and drink a cup of tea. Heinrich was slightly mollified when a cup was handed to him. I was taken back to prison without the slightest chance of escape. It was a scatterbrained attempt but in desperate times even the wise man will rush in.

The escapade was over. The guards accepted the cut as an accident, although Heinrich retained some suspicions, for he was later to tell me that if I had made an attempt to escape he would have shot me. In telling this, he tapped the pistol hanging from his belt. I was now back in the dreariness of prison life. My only reward for a cut arm was some very old magazines and a book the nurses had given me. Heinrich, of course, searched them for files or a machine gun before they could be handed to me. He was a morose man with no joy whatsoever. The nurses had been pretty, cheerful girls deserving some admiration. I had flirted in between winces as the needle went in and out but Heinrich, except for demands for silence, stood stony faced throughout.

Life dribbled on, Christmas came and on Christmas Day we were allowed to see our near relatives. My whole family came to visit. They had brought me a small parcel which contained a nice piece of cake which I thought owed a lot to Denis. They were all unhappy and my younger sister was in tears. However, they found me cheerful. The well informed grapevine of the prison assured me that it would all soon be over.

My cheerfulness spread and when I called to Otto and introduced him as 'Otto, the Punch nosed, pot bellied son of the devil,' smiling at him in good fellowship and, as far as his English went, I was praising his good German attributes. Everyone smiled. We talked as we wished, there was little to hear from home, my father whispered that it was almost over and I thought that one of my crystal sets had avoided detection and was still in use. I told them that prison was not that bad, many friends were there. My request to Otto to be allowed to visit him in prison next Christmas ended the visit.

My second attempt at escape was very nearly successful and only the cruel fates in the shape of two local guards prevented success. Early in January, 1945, an excellent plan was made possible by the good offices of a youth proficient in the use of picklocks. Douglas the picklock! The centre cells on both floors were different from all the others in that their doors could be opened from the inside as, unlike all the others, the lock extended through the door with a keyhole on either side.

I was given to understand that these two cells were for naughty guards who could lock themselves in and let themselves out when their time was up. Douglas, with two others, occupied the centre cell on the ground floor and, with a simple piece of curved metal, he opened his cell door and roamed the corridor as he pleased. With great glee, he would tap on one or another of the cell doors and chat with its occupants. He could also, using the same implement, open any of the cell doors from the outside. He made no other use of this freedom of movement within the cell block but I thought it had possibilities.

On one of the morning exercises, I asked Douglas if he could open my door so that I could have a look at a store room at the east end of the corridor. He was happy to oblige and immediately after our noon mug of swill when the guards were most unlikely to be seen until the afternoon exercise three hours later, Douglas opened my cell door and the two of us went to examine the store. The door was locked but Douglas was able to unlock and open it in seconds. The store in itself was of no interest, however, the door in its far north end was, for unlocking it we discovered that it gave access to a long narrow yard, one wall being the cell block wall, the other was a ten foot high granite wall, the other side of which was the paved entry area from the main gate. A perfect escape route, for once over this ten foot wall the only obstacle would be the main prison gate attended by local Jersey guards.

Escape would have been a simple matter, except that Douglas did not wish to escape. Neither did he wish the guard to know that he had been instrumental in the escape. We returned to our cells and my next twenty four hours was given to thinking of an escape for which only the escapee could be blamed. Bubble, bubble, toil and trouble, remove the toil and trouble The answer was simple - block up the door keep with cardboard, when the spring lock catch on the cell door would not lock into position and the door could be opened from inside my cell. This, in fact, did not work as the power of the spring lock always compressed whatever was packed into the keep. I knew this very well for I had tried it on more than one occasion. However, the guards would not know that it did not work, the evidence of a stuffed keep would be more than enough for them. So it proved to be.

Two days after our reconnaissance, I declined the morning exercise and made my preparation. Declining exercise was common as it was the only way to take a bath in private. The bathing was a bucket of water, cold and a piece of cloth with which one mopped oneself down. My preparations were to cut pieces of cardboard into strips and be ready to jam these pieces into the keep when exercise was over and soup was being distributed. Cell doors were open for three or four minutes during this period. Declining exercise was not really necessary as I could have prepared the cardboard at any time but Germans like a bit of planning and if they could not trace the plan leading to the execution, they might well be suspicious.

The door, of course, locked. The cardboard did not work but Douglas was to hand. My two cell mates refused the chance of escape as did all the cell occupants. A great shame really for we could have had a mass breakout which would have been tremendous fun and a great victory over our enemies. Douglas came, opened my door and the two doors to the store. If caught, I would say that the first was open and the door into the yard I had opened with a bent rusty nail which was purposely left on the floor near the yard door.

Giving Douglas a few minutes to return to his cell, I carried the store bench into the yard which I placed against the external wall, went back for a steel box - rather like a small cabin trunk - which I placed on the table. Climbing on these two, I was able to look over the wall. All was clear, so I climbed over and dropped into the main prison entrance yard. The main gates where two Jersey guards, Atropos and Clotho (Lachesis was on holiday) were on duty, was fifteen yards away but all was lost!

These guards, seeing me climb over the wall and drop to the ground in their area, had pressed the alarm bell. If they had immediately opened the gate as I asked - demanded would be a better word - I might still have made good my escape but they firmly refused. They were not armed and a trial of strength crossed my mind. I waited too long as the idea of attacking one's own made me hesitant. The alarm bell must have had major importance for it sounded in both the local prison and the German prison.

Two local guards came running, immediately followed by Heinrich and Otto. The local guards unarmed and Heinrich and Otto both with their pistols in their hands. The two local main entrance guards seemed proud of their achievement but a few months after the end of the Occupation, one of them called at my parents house with profuse apologies, his excuse being that he and his companion would have been in the most serious trouble had they let me go.

I was out at the time, had I been at home, I do not think I would have forgiven them as they should have taken their chances, as we all did in those days. Some arrangement and story could have been concocted.

I was taken back to the German prison by Heinrich and Otto, the former white with anger, the latter, bright red and sweating. Heinrich screamed that I had made fools of them. But he was wrong, they had been fools long before I came on the scene. I was beyond fear, filled with regret that my excellent plan had failed. I therefore voiced my opinion of both of them and received a blow to the side of my head from Heinrich's pistol. Otto would dearly have wished to do the same but my anger at the blow to the head must have appeared on my face: he was now more than ever cautious of me.

However, they still pushed and prodded me with their pistols, Otto tentatively, until we were safely in the German compound. Cheffy joined in the great pantomime of outraged German pride. He could not show his concern and anger nearly enough and skips and dances accompanied his tirade. I was not beaten but as outrage ebbed and flowed, I was pushed again and again.

My method of escape was explained, the packed cardboard door keep examined, the bent nail on the floor of the store room near the yard door was discovered with idiotic triumph. My cell mates were questioned. They said that they were asleep when I slipped out, which, believe it or not, the trio of guards had little option but to accept. There was no conspiracy and I was entirely to blame. With such possessions as I had, I was searched once again for files or machine guns, taken across to the German prisoners cell block and there placed in solitary confinement. I do not think that the escape was reported to the Gestapo as I saw nothing of Karl.

With all their German efficiency - which in my firm opinion is mythical - they had made a fatal mistake for I was located in cell no.2. Immediately next door, in cell number 1, was Don Bell and Frank Le Pennec and escape number three was in the planning stage almost the moment I was locked in my cell. Communication with Don and Frank was possible during the following days exercise periods where up and down the ninety yards of rough pavement, the first plan outline was hewn and, on later exercise periods, refined and polished to our great satisfaction.

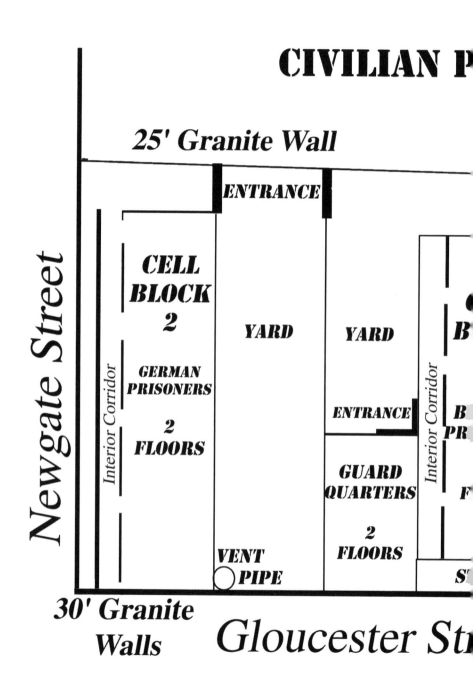

CIVILIAN P

25' Granite Wall

ENTRANCE

Newgate Street

Interior Corridor

CELL
BLOCK
2

GERMAN
PRISONERS

2
FLOORS

YARD

YARD

ENTRANCE

GUARD
QUARTERS

2
FLOORS

Interior Corridor

B

B
PR

F

VENT
PIPE

S

30' Granite
Walls

Gloucester St

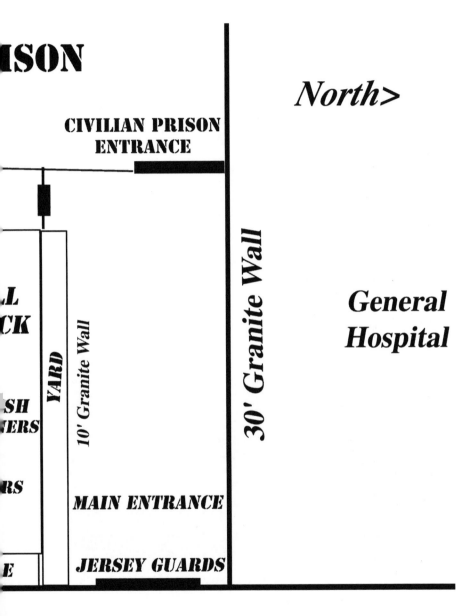

ISON

North>

**CIVILIAN PRISON
ENTRANCE**

30' Granite Wall

General
Hospital

L
CK

YARD

10' Granite Wall

SH
ERS

RS

MAIN ENTRANCE

E

JERSEY GUARDS

et

Main Prison Entrance

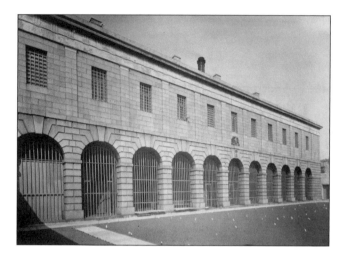

Yard

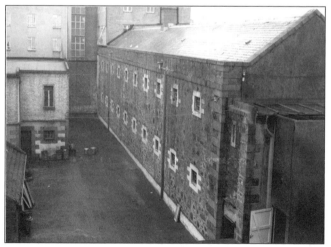

From right to left lower. First cell window, Don and Frank
Second cell window, me.

Corridor

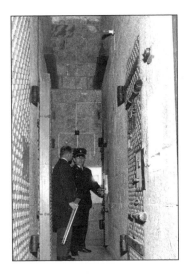

Cell

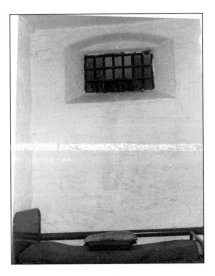

CHAPTER 11
ESCAPE

The German prisoners cell block was to the south of the German complex. It was an old building and more than likely dated from Victorian times. It was built entirely of granite blocks, was cold, very damp, entirely forbidding and may well have been the end of the line in days past. My cell, in accoutrements was exactly similar to my previous cell but with a black steel door rather than grey and the window, due to the granite walls being twice as thick, appeared much smaller. The floors were also of granite and the building faced north so that sunlight never entered the cells.

The guards were different, except for Cheffy who made his appearance from time to time. These guards were soldiers, not professional guards and possibly for that reason were better men than Heinrich and Otto. Therefore any regret in making an escape would be the punishment meted out to the guard on duty on the escape night. There were four of them, two being young men not above twenty, the other two, worn out old soldiers.

There were in excess of one hundred German prisoners of whom we saw very little as our exercise periods were different to theirs and the height of the window from the cell floor made it very difficult to peer at them during their exercise periods.

Frank Le Pennec and Don Bell were in the first cell on the left on entering the cell block and I was immediately next door, both cells being next to the entrance at the far western end of the block with the long line of cell windows on two levels facing on to the exercise yard. This yard running east to west was entirely surrounded by granite walls or buildings. To the east, a thirty feet high granite wall on Gloucester Street, the west wall of similar height and construction separated the civilian prison from the German prison. The north wall partly enclosed the guards quarters, windowless on that elevation and of course the south elevation was our cell block which was built against another thirty feet high granite wall on Newgate Street, the cell block being some five feet lower than the Newgate Street wall it was built against. There was a twenty five feet vent pipe encased with barbed wire in the far south corner, built against the cell block.

Why Don and Frank were lodged in the German prisoners section of the prison, I do not know, however, they must have done something bad. The very next morning after my arrival we were together at exercise and discussed events since we had last seen each other. I described my escape attempt and we immediately discussed an attempt of our own and thereafter we talked of little else. Our plans were quick to materialise as on 12th. February, 1945 we made our escape.

To succeed, our plan depended heavily on the naïveté of one or other of the two young guards and because of his good nature and almost childish innocence, the younger, Walter, was chosen to be the sacrificial lamb. We easily obtained a section of angle iron from the supports of cables and pipes running along the corridor. The piece chosen had been welded together in an L shape and we thought it would do for a grapnel. Lengths of blankets were cut to form a rope which required trial and error as the blankets available were old and tended to break under test.

These tests and most of this work was carried out by Don and Frank by securing one end of the cut blanket to the cell window grill and the two of them pulling with all their might. The idea was to gain entry to the yard, throw the grapnel over the roof of the cell block, gain a hold and climb up, using the rope and grapnel for the decent into Newgate Street. After two hundred and seventy circuits of the exercise yard, all preparations were complete, the plan was put into action. With Walter on duty, we moved at around 8pm on a dry February night.

For five days I had returned to my cell after exercise with a chamber pot filled with water to pour it in the corner of my cell below a water pipe running along the wall under the window. The cell floor sloped enough for the water to pond under the pipe and give a first impression of a badly leaking pipe. This initial part of the escape plan worked perfectly. Don or Frank rang an alarm bell which was located in each cell and rang in the guards quarters. The guard on duty would come to see and deal with whatever was the cause for the alarm to be used.

Walter came, unlocked but did not lock behind him the main door, went to Don and Frank's cell where they excitedly told him that there was something wrong with me. Poor Walter fitted exactly into the part we had planned, hoped and expected of him. He did not lock Don and Frank in their cells but, accompanied by them, he came to my cell, unlocked the door and saw me in great distress, pointing to the pool of water under the window. He stared, noticed the water then went forward for a close look. I pushed him in the back, ran out of the cell and slammed the door shut. Walter had no way out as there was no keyhole on the inside. We tore down electrical cables running along the corridor to stop the use of the emergency bell and gained the yard. Perfect planning and perfect execution until outside in the yard the plan went badly wrong.

The grapnel would not work. We could not throw it to the roof parapet as, together with the blanket rope it was too heavy. Worse still, Walter was shouting for blue murder through the window of my cell and very soon all the German prisoners were joining in. We had no choice but to run to the vent pipe in the far corner for guards were coming from the guards quarters and we had to climb the barbed wire vent pipe with bare hands. Presumably the barbed wire had been wrapped around the pipe to prevent what we were now doing but without the barbed wire we could not have climbed the pipe.

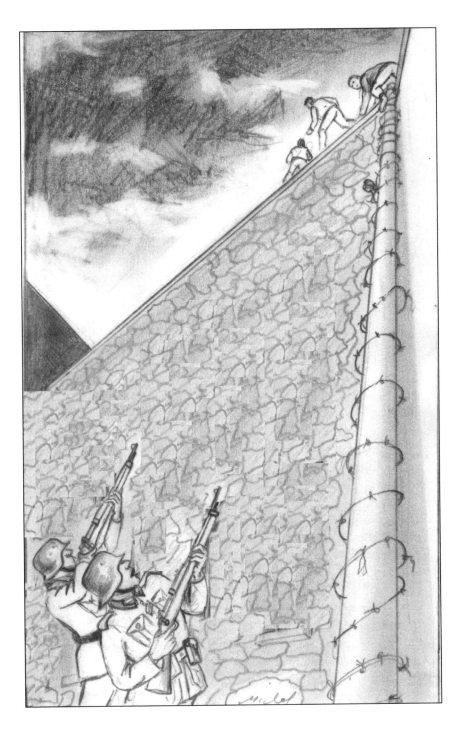

I felt no pain as I climbed, the desperation of the moment was an absolute anaesthetic. Pain was to come later. Don went first, followed by Frank and I brought up the rear. We clambered up like monkeys, clothing was torn and I lost one shoe in the barbed wire. Before I reached the top the guards appeared, questions and answers exchanged, shots were fired, indiscriminately at first, as it was dark and they fired in our general direction. We had all cleared the vent pipe and were on the prison roof by the time they reached the foot of the pipe and fired in anger as their quarry were out of sight. It was truly a famous event, the guards yelling, guns firing, all the German prisoners in a frenzy of excitement, the whole prison complex aware something momentous had occurred.

I was later to be told that rumours among the prisoners were rampant in the following days. We had all been shot, one had been shot, we had escaped and so on. We crossed the roof to the external wall and faced a drop into Newgate Street, thirty feet below. Don jumped, followed by Frank, I climbed up on the wall, hung at arms length, prayed, let go and dropped. I did not hit the pavement, it came up and hit me with great force and I was unable to move for many seconds. I had fallen correctly, squarely on both feet but the ankle of my shoeless left foot was broken. Both Don and Frank had gone and, as we had never given much thought as to where we should find refuge in planning the escape, I limped off in aimless panic. I made my way through the back streets through the park and reached the top of Westmount. My ankle was swollen and would no longer take my weight. I was covered in blood from torn hands and legs, the front of my trousers having been torn to shreds by the barbed wire. I was and looked a mess.

I sat on the grass by the side of the road and asked people returning home before curfew to help me but on the explanation that I had escaped from the German prison, they were too frightened to offer assistance. They may have also had worries about my physical condition for, although the cuts were superficial, I was covered in blood and as far as they were concerned, I may have had a fatal wound. There were not that many people about and my appeal was made to five or six without success. A young couple would have helped, if they had dared, as they stayed for some time, compassionate but indecisive. They were frightened, the young woman plainly terrified. The husband, a potential good samaritan, reluctantly left, dragged by his wife leaving the world to darkness and to me. Curfew time was near when only German patrols would be abroad. I supposed that I had spent three hours sitting on the grass when a German patrol picked me up. To give these two soldiers all credit, they spent little time in questions. One left and the other stayed with me. Within fifteen minutes the guard returned with two soldiers, a stretcher and an officer. They placed me on a stretcher and carried me on up the hill to a German occupied house, which must have been a first aid station because I was taken to a room lined with hospital beds.

The two soldier stretcher bearers were just about to lift me off the stretcher on to one of these beds when the officer stopped them. His reasoning must have been that I was bloody and would stain the blanket. It soon developed that he was fully aware of who I was as they were on the alert for escaped prisoners and only wasted his time on the minimum of questions.

He sent one of the orderlies for help and Brunnhilde appeared, 'Sometimes it isn't half as bad as all that, sometimes.' Brunnhilde was tall, statuesque, bluest of blue eyes and golden hair plaited around her head with loose tendrils kissing her pink cheeks. Brunnhilde was a nurse. She gave her instructions, lost the argument of my being put on the bed but won a concession as one of orderlies left and returned with a blanket, not new but clean and thick, waited until warm water was brought in, then knelt on the floor by the stretcher and washed my hands, wrists and shins.

She noted the numerous cuts and questioned the officer. At his reply, she looked at me with both surprise and curiosity but continued her gentle nursing. She examined my ankle, gently touching and moving it about and again asked questions of the officer. On his reply, she placed

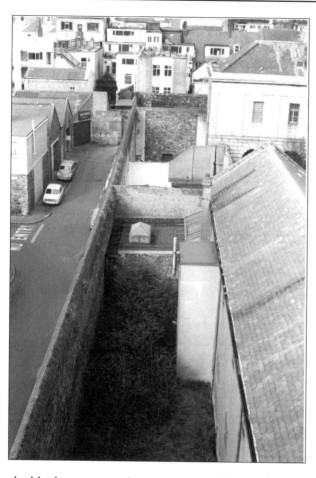

Our jump into
Newgate Street.

the blanket over me then sat on one of the beds looking at me and the officer. The two orderlies remained standing, also looking down at me. There was rather a helpless look on the faces of the stretcher bearers, commiseration from Brunnhilde and just a look from the officer.

This lasted for thirty minutes or more until another officer arrived. He asked me if I was one of the escaped prisoners, I said yes, as there was little to gain from a denial. He then asked where my two friends were and my answer that I did not know caused him to shout angry questions at the first officer who, by his heightened complexion, was unable to acknowledge that any search for my two friends was ordered by him. However, on further questioning and satisfied that we had gone our separate ways after the escape, he calmed down.

Orders were given to the stretcher bearers and I was taken to and placed in an ambulance which had been parked outside. I was carried from the ward. I managed a great smile and wave to Brunnhilde. Perhaps her real name was Cora?

I was taken back to prison and back to my cell which I had left some seven hours before. Both Heinrich and Otto guided my two stretcher bearers to my cell and watched as I was placed on the wooden bed. They were both very subdued. Defeat, I think, had at last caught up with them. The door was locked and I was alone but not for long, the key was heard in the lock, the door thrown open and Cheffy entered.

He was incoherent with rage, spluttering and gesticulating waving a metal soup ladle. It must have been the nearest object to hand when he had left the guards quarters. With cries of rage he beat me with the ladle which, owing to his anger, missed me more often than he hit me. However, by the time he left, two broken or cracked ribs were added to my other injuries. Although sore and aching, I was very tired and fell asleep. My only consolation was Brunnhilde and I had gained a nice warm, thick blanket.

Next morning Cheffy called and told me that a doctor would soon come to see me. He then asked me not to tell anyone of the soup ladle incident of the night before. This request was a plea and I promised my silence in the hope of better treatment in the future, thinking that this particular bird was better than two unknowns in the bushes.

A German doctor followed soon after, accompanied by a medical orderly. The doctor satisfied himself that there was nothing very wrong with me and left me within ten minutes under the care of the orderly.

This uniformed orderly was a very good man, he fussed, talked soothingly, strapped my ribs with a tight bandage, applied some sort of antiseptic cream to the cuts on my legs and hands and, after much pressing and moving of my left foot and ankle, now swollen and an angry red, he said that it was not broken and was better left as it was for the time being as an X-ray was necessary. He would return that evening.

He is remembered largely because of a birthmark covering the whole of the left side of his face. The X-ray never happened but he attended me with great care and kindness for three weeks.

Later that day a youth, Joe Mière, was sent to share my cell and look after me. Poor Joe had his work cut out as I could not walk without assistance and had to be half carried to and from the usual offices. Joe looked after me with great kindness and although I must assume that I thanked him then, I again thank him now. Joe's kindness went beyond normal limits. He had been a hairdresser before his imprisonment. He had a comb and pair of scissors and kindly cut my hair some six or seven times in as many weeks until, sadly for Joe, there was no hair left to cut.

Of course the Gestapo came. Karl arrived the very morning after the escape, he wanted to know where Don and Frank were. I was able to convince him that none of us knew what we should do once on the outside but were prepared to try our luck. My own aimless wandering tended to prove my statement. Don's mother was imprisoned for a few weeks in an attempt to entice him back but this failed as Don never knew that his mother was imprisoned. Don had found refuge with friends, who had taken him to a doctor's residence in the country where he stayed throughout the remainder of the Occupation. Frank's refuge was so simple and unexpected that the Gestapo had not the slightest suspicion. He went home!

Karl called very often over the following weeks. His visits became social and we discussed poetry, both English and German, the law and its interpretation in both countries. I had little or no knowledge of law but listened. Karl had been a law student before the Nazis caught up with him. In 1930 he would have been twenty five and his knowledge appeared to be pre-Hitler. He was also very interested in the British political system. Again I knew very little. Listening, one became aware that Karl had political ambitions and if he spoke as he felt, democracy was in his mind. He asked for no favours and I offered none. However, I told him that when questioned by British Intelligence, I would tell the truth. He said that he would be happy if I did so.

In these various discussions he told me that we were lucky that we had not been caught six months before, as we would certainly have been sent to Germany and a prison camp. He was not an evil man: none of them were but they were working amid and surrounded by evil, it would be difficult to cleanse themselves. However, I supposed that Germans are like sponges and absorbed the prevailing fashion.

I asked Karl why did he not let us go? He said that he could not, as he was still subject to orders. He also explained that he was not in the Gestapo but in Operational Field Police of some sort. He appeared uncomfortable with my questions on his always being dressed in civilian dress and, in British eyes, was a Music Hall act as to how the Gestapo were meant to look.

The last two months of the Occupation lingered on with little to break the monotony. Red Cross food parcels had arrived in late February so that the prison food was no longer of any hardship. The boredom, cold, damp and our old friends Otto, Heinrich and Cheffy remained. I told Otto that the British had plans to hang him for being fat whilst all his prisoners were half starved. I pointed to his pot belly as I spoke and made motions of the noose being hung about his neck. As far as he understood, it was a good British joke and he laughed for ten minutes.

Heinrich was more morose than ever. Cheffy ran around trying to please everyone. They were clockwork soldiers all: they travelled their well known path but little more. I really needed a plan of escape to break the boredom but that would have been the stupidest thing I had ever done for clockwork soldiers drew their pistols and fired, albeit in a clockwork fashion.

I never thought of the simplest plan, demand to be released or otherwise tell the British great lies of torture, beatings and horrible atrocities. It might have worked with Otto and Cheffy, particularly the latter as I had something on him. Walter still lived for I saw him looking through his cell window. I called to him - 'Good old Walter! You will soon be free!' He smiled, though I doubt that he understood me.

At around noon on a fine spring morning I was surprised, astonished and full of hopeful expectation, in that order. Gracie Fields was singing, the sound coming from the direction of the Opera House, over the wall and across the road from the prison. Her song? Look up and laugh and laugh your troubles away . It proved to be correct as a loudspeaker had been attached to the external wall of the Opera House blaring out records broadcast for us to hear. Less than an hour later the cell doors were flung open by British soldiers come to our rescue. We were free!

Freedom was a little of an anticlimax at first, I had been imprisoned for over seven months. I did not go straight home but wandered into the Royal Square where a great crowd had gathered. I stood on the fringes and listened to their merriment. Joy was unconfined and the feeling of something good having happened entered my being. My last German adventure then occurred. A drunken German officer approached the fringes of the crowd almost exactly next to me, brandished a pistol and shouting, in English, that he was going to shoot someone, that Germany was not defeated.

With the help of two men he was disarmed. The pistol, in fact, was not loaded. He put up very little resistance and I must pay great praise and respect for the people in the immediate vicinity for they showed no thoughts of revenge. They patted him on the back and told him to be a good German. As I left I saw him with a group of people singing happily along with them. The pistol? One of the two men with me must have kept it as a souvenir.

I went home and whereas there was welcome and pleasure at my return, there was also anxiety. Contact with Britain had been restored but there was no telephone in the house and means of communication were by telegrams and letters. My parents were desperately in search of news of my elder brother, Middy. News came four days after liberation. Middy had been killed in action in Hong Kong in December, 1941. Liberation was of secondary importance, Middy was in everyone's mind. My poor mother, on hearing the news, immediately left the house and was not seen again for eight or nine hours. She had wandered aimlessly with her misery. It would be months before she could be tolerably content and weeks before any degree of cheerfulness returned to the house.

I was interviewed by British Intelligence and, with a sergeant, was taken back to the prison on two different occasions. I found that the Gestapo were imprisoned in the same cell-block where I had spent the latter part of my imprisonment. Both Karl and Wolf were there with four of the lesser members of their group. I identified them all and told my story. They were very interested in the 'observer' during my questioning at Gestapo Headquarters but he was not there.

All the Gestapo were now in uniform, posing as Field Police or perhaps they had posed as Gestapo in the first place. Karl was sullen. He did communicate when questioned by the sergeant. I told Karl, that, as I had promised, I had made a true statement for which the intelligence officer had been pleased, as they had received many conflicting stories of beatings. The Intelligence sergeant told me that Karl had become of interest to them, mainly due to the conflicting reports of his conduct during the Occupation and his political ideas. I had reported Karl's various conversations with me.

In questioning by the Intelligence sergeant, I had been asked if I had been treated well by any Germans during my imprisonment. I told of Brunnhilde, the medical orderly with the birthmark and the old crippled soldier at Gestapo headquarters. They asked for names and rank - which I could not give them. Their purpose was early release for proven good Germans. My descriptions were enough, they said, as a medical orderly with a birthmark would not be difficult to find. Karl could help them with the old soldier and German nurses were not likely to be long detained. I hope that Brunnhilde finds Siegfried, the medical orderly finds Sara and the Old Soldier fades away in comfort and peace.

The summer of 1945 was to see the break-up of the pool crowd. There were many outside interests and activities and the pool was no longer the haven it had been during the long years of the Occupation. During that summer I found work with the British army, guarding arms and explosives stored at Longueville Manor. I was now amidst all the objects I had once coveted and although there was much to interest me, I coveted none.

There were six of us and our main job was to keep children away from the many dangerous objects stored there. The first hectic weeks of the Liberation over, life returned to normal or I supposed that it had. Insofar as the latter third of my life had seemed normal to me, I was unsure and would require time to appreciate normality.

CHAPTER 12
AND SO IT WAS

In early autumn I was planning to travel to England - which would be an adventure as previously I had never travelled anywhere but Jersey and Guernsey. I first went to Bournemouth where I stayed for a few weeks with an aunt and uncle, then moved to London. I joined the R.A.F. and in February of the following year I was in India where I found neither tigers nor an Indian princess. I had exchanged one form of regimentation for another but, of course, one was much more benign than the other.

Before leaving Jersey I paid a last visit to the dip in the hill, near the lodge on the road to Rozel. I leaned on the railings under the trees where Stephanie had often waited for me so long ago. I had no real expectations but an ember of hope faintly glowed. I imagined that she would come, a young woman now. We would meet and her lovely smile would light up her face, altogether beautiful. Night birds called, the cold fingers of approaching winter touched my cheek, darkness came but never Stephanie.

So it was!

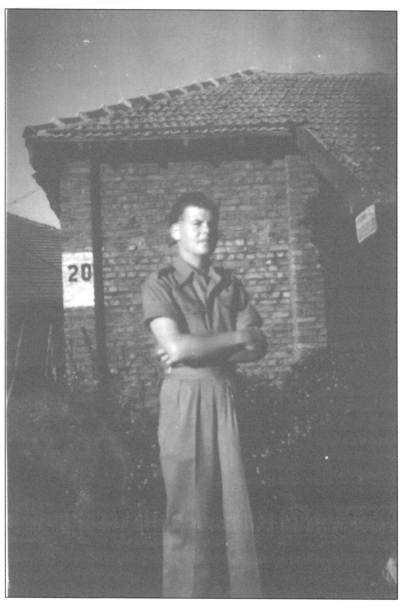

Me as a young man in 1945

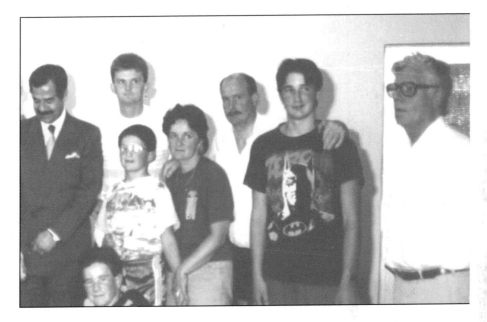

Here I am pictured with Saddam Hussein

Saddam far left, me far right

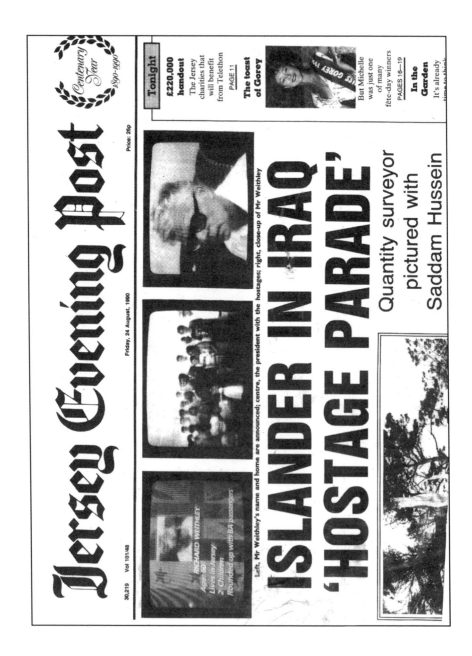

Jersey Evening Post

Centenary Year 1890–1990

30,219   Vol 101/148   Friday, 24 August, 1990   Price: 25p

Tonight

£220,000 handout

The Jersey charities that will benefit from Teletbon

PAGE 11

The toast of Gorey

But Michelle was just one of many fête-day winners

PAGES 16–19

In the Garden

It's already time to think

ISLANDER IN IRAQ 'HOSTAGE PARADE'

Quantity surveyor pictured with Saddam Hussein

Left, Mr Weithley's name and home are announced; centre, the president with the hostages; right, close-up of Mr Weithley

RICHARD WEITHLEY
Age: 60
Lives in Jersey
2 Children
Rounded up with BA passengers

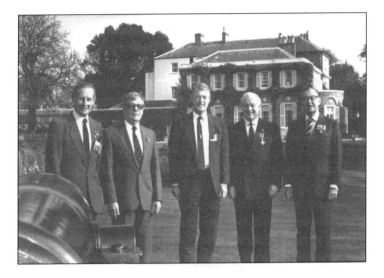

Me at Government House on my return from Iraq.

Key Map of Events

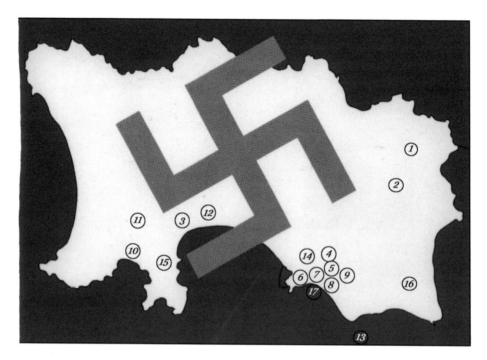

The following locations in the book are situated in St Helier:
Prison
Commercial Street Store
Esplanade (Capture)
Grand Hotel
Beaufort Hotel
Colomberie Hotel
West's Cinema
Europa Hotel

1) Rozel
2) Stephanie's House (St Martin)
3) Colonel Swan (Beaumont)
4) Beeches
5) Merton Hotel Armoury
6) South Pier Gun Bunker
7) Green Street Gun Bunker
8) Gestapo Headquarters (Havre des Pas)
9) St Luke's German Store
10) Tams Pantry- (Floats St Brelade)
11) German rail line (Red Houses)
12) Goose Green (Russian camp, Beaumont)
13) Shipwreck (Demi des Pas)
14) Westmount (Escape route)
15) Ghost Hill (Wooden Guns, St Aubin)
16) Joe's Farm (Grouville)
17) The Pool & Flour Store (Havre des Pas)

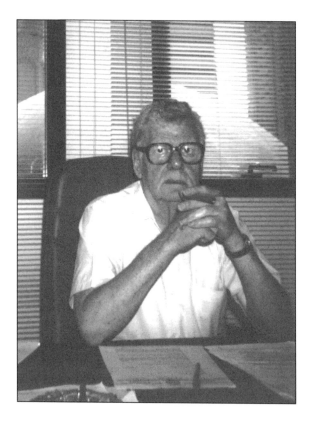

About the Author

The author was born in Guernsey in April 1926, moved to - or was moved - to Jersey in 1928 where he now resides. Leaving Jersey in 1946, he enlisted in the R.A.F and spent most of 1946 through 1949 in India. He witnessed and was partly involved in the racial riots of 1946 in that country. Returning to England in 1950 he joined a professional quantity surveying practice located in London.

He has travelled extensively in his profession, working in Gibraltar, Kuwait, Lebanon, United Arab Emirates, Yemen, Oman, Egypt, West Indies and Albania. As senior partner of 'L.R Weithley and Associates (Jersey) Ltd' he is presently employed in Kuwait, Cairo and Albania.

His only claim to fame is imprisonment by courtesy of the Germans in 1944 - 1945, and by courtesy of Saddam Hussein, Iraq - August 1990 to December 1990.

He is married and has two children resident in Jersey and Spain.

His reason for writing this book, or so he claims, may be self evident. The Occupation of Jersey was not all doom and gloom and certainly Jersey folk were by no means collaborators.

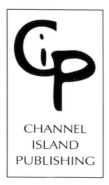

CHANNEL
ISLAND
PUBLISHING

Other Occupation titles from Channel Island Publishing...

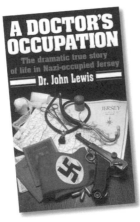

A Doctor's Occupation
First published in 1982 by
Transworld Publishers, this well
known Occupation book, published
locally from 1997, is still a firm
favourite.

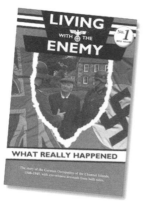

Living With The Enemy
Published in 1995, this book about
the German Occupation of the
Channel Islands has hit the No.1
spot every year as the best-selling
local book.

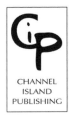

CHANNEL
ISLAND
PUBLISHING

Channel Island Publishing

Other titles from the same publisher

LIVING WITH THE ENEMY
A DOCTOR'S OCCUPATION
THE ISLANDS' RICH & FAMOUS
GLANCE BACK IN AMAZEMENT
HITLER'S BRITISH ISLANDS
TWO FLAGS ONE HEART
TOUJOURS JEUNE
JERSEY: ISLE OF AVALON
THE OPERA HOUSE JERSEY
MONT ORGUEIL CASTLE A SOUVENIR GUIDE
THE ISLAND OF JERSEY VIDEO SOUVENIR
THE ISLAND OF GUERNSEY VIDEO SOUVENIR
HISTORICAL LINKS: HISTORY OF THE ROYAL JERSEY GOLF CLUB

FOR DETAILS OF THESE AND MANY OTHER
BOOKS VISIT OUR WEBSITE
www.channelislandpublishing.com

Channel Island Publishing
UNIT 3B, BARETTE COMMERCIAL CENTRE
LA ROUTE DU MONT MADO
ST.JOHN, JERSEY, CHANNEL ISLANDS, JE3 4DS
TEL 44 (0) 1534 860806 FAX 44 (0) 1534 860811
E-MAIL sales@channelislandpublishing,com